THE MAN

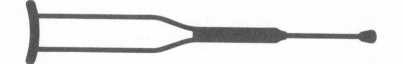

WHO LEARNED

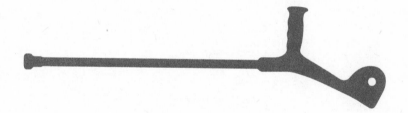

TO WALK

THREE TIMES

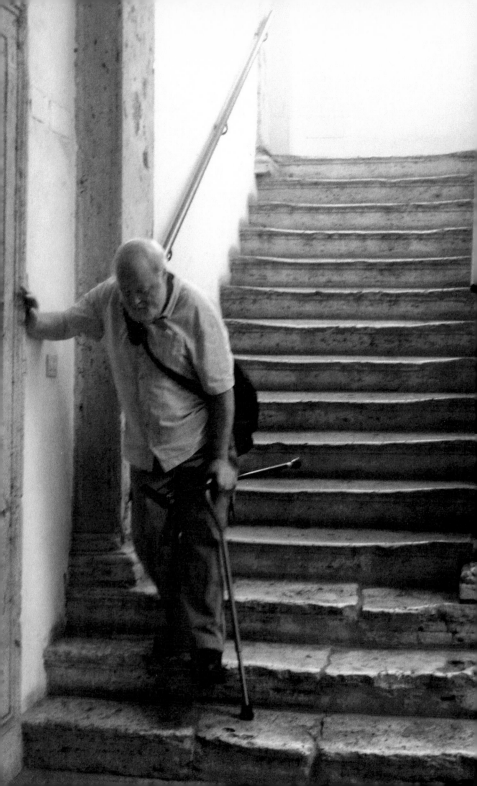

THE
MAN
WHO
LEARNED
TO
WALK
THREE
TIMES

A MEMOIR

PETER
KAVANAGH

Alfred A. Knopf Canada

PUBLISHED BY ALFRED A. KNOPF CANADA

www.penguinrandomhouse.ca

Knopf Canada and colophon are registered trademarks.

Library and Archives Canada Cataloguing in Publication

Kavanagh, Peter, 1953–, author
    The man who learned to walk three times : a memoir / Peter Kavanagh.

Issued in print and electronic formats.

ISBN 978-0-345-80852-3
eBook ISBN 978-0-345-80854-7

    1. Kavanagh, Peter, 1953––Health. 2. Kavanagh, Peter, 1953–. 3. Poliomyelitis—
Psychological aspects. 4. Poliomyelitis—Patients—Rehabilitation—Canada.
5. Poliomyelitis—Patients—Canada—Biography. 6. Journalists—Canada—Biography.
I. Title.

RC181.C2K39 2015   362.196'8350092   C2014-906375-X

Book design by Andrew Roberts

Family snapshots courtesy of the author.
Cover photo and all other photos by Debi Goodwin.
Interior images: (cane and crutches) © Dece11 / Dreamstime.com

Printed and bound in the United States of America

10 9 8 7 6 5 4 3 2 1

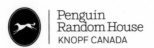

Penguin
Random House
KNOPF CANADA

For my parents,
who were there for the first two times
I learned to walk but missed the third.

CONTENTS

PART THREE

PREFACE

I n September 2013, I travelled to Italy. Within an hour of arriving, I was climbing up old marble steps that had become pitted and worn over the centuries. Using my cane and an iron handrail bolted into the wall, I found a spot on the uneven and slippery surface where I could position myself to move my right leg to the next step, and then my left. There were two flights of fifteen steps each between the courtyard of the ancient building in Rome's Jewish ghetto and the landing leading to the apartment we'd rented. Going up, I would stop at each step, take a breath and think about how to position myself so as to step up most efficiently, with the emphasis on moving my body primarily through my legs. Going down, I would stop, take a breath and calculate how best to position myself so as to step down without falling while at the same time moving as quickly as possible. Going up and going down, I would feel a certain self-mocking frustration. The only thing that irritated me more than these stairs was trying to sort through the set of five keys necessary to unlock the various doors between the street and our temporary home.

Several times a day for the next four days, that was the routine. It wore out my body, worried at my mind and oddly exhilarated me. I was petrified that I would lose my footing, fall and injure myself, and ultimately become even more of a burden than I already was. I was equally certain that everyone was watching me and laughing at my clear ineptitude at this most basic of tasks.

At the same time, I wanted and needed to do this trip. When I booked the apartment, I had no idea about the stairs and what simply going in and out might entail, and when I first saw the steps I felt a momentary panic but then kept going. This is what people do—struggle with difficulty and move on. I was thinking, if I can do this, even clumsily and with great effort, what else can I do?

The next several weeks in Italy were filled with cobblestone, uneven pavement and sloping piazzas. Sometimes I could not surmount these challenges. Other times, obstacles that would have paralyzed me into inaction even six months earlier seemed like nothing.

For three weeks, I walked up and down slopes that terrified me; worked muscles, tendons and joints in ways they had never been worked before; experienced new types of pain and fatigue; and thought about the walking I had just done, the walking I would do tomorrow and whether I would ever be able to stop thinking about walking.

Walking is the key to who I am.

How I walk today, the canes and walking sticks I have owned, the braces I have worn and wear, the shoes I can't buy, the shoes I can, how I think about my walking, how other people think of my walking—all have been ravelled together and constitute the heart of me.

My earliest memories, stark images of figures in masks wrapping me in restrictive cloth; my recent dreams of moving, being unable to move, of standing and falling (varying in frequency, detail, and degree of terror and joy); my most common flashbacks; my aversion to mirrors and plate glass windows; my formerly constant speculating about how people perceived my limp—this entire maze and mess of interior dialogue is the cause and consequence of a lifelong and unusual attention to walking. And a lifelong attention to walking is not normal.

The *Oxford English Dictionary* defines walking as "mov[ing] at a regular pace by lifting and setting down each foot in turn, never having both feet off the ground at once." Seems simple, even straightforward. The OED could have gone on to note that walking is one of the key "unconscious" activities that human beings do. We learn how to walk and then simply do it, with little thought. K.H. Thomann, a renowned expert in normal and abnormal walking, wrote, "For most people, walking is an automatic, unconscious activity, characteristic of each individual. . . . Most parents who watch an infant beginning to walk realize that locomotion is a highly complex, learned process. Years of training and practice are necessary for the sensory-motor system to become adept at automatically generating the motor commands necessary to permit walking without conscious effort."

Saint Denis, the patron saint of walkers, was killed in 250 CE by beheading. The story goes that he then picked up his head and carried it for almost ten kilometres, preaching all the way. The legend displays an essential understanding of the science and practice of walking, which is much more about tissue, nerve, muscle, tendon, habit and experience than it is about conscious thought. Putting aside the question of the miraculous, if you can deliver a sermon while carrying your own head and walking, then clearly the power of unconscious activities enables and supports the most basic of human multi-tasking.

On that trip to Italy, which was both a holiday and an experiment, the constant attention I paid to my walking caused every muscle to tense up and, over the course of a day, wore me out mentally and physically. I was the guy who slowed traffic and disrupted the flow of pedestrians. I can't count the number of vistas, odd occurrences and magnificent buildings and sculptures that I missed because I was concentrating on navigating a particular piece of cobblestone or a missing piece of pavement.

Getting walking right is learning not to think about it. That is almost the definition of what it means to learn to walk. It is a lesson I have learned three times.

PART

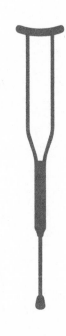

ONE

1

A PLAGUE

I was born near the deepest waters of the Ottawa River, in a town and at a time when cutting-edge science and widespread panic about an old medical plague lived side by side. In 1614, the explorer Samuel de Champlain declared the river bottomless in this spot, but we now know that the current just drags the measuring device along so slowly that it feels as though it hasn't touched bottom. The town built here—Deep River, Ontario, two hundred kilometres northwest of Ottawa—was created in 1944 as part of the Manhattan Project. It was designed to be the living quarters of the group of people associated with Canada's nuclear programme and the proposed nuclear facility at Chalk River, just down the road. The men (for they were mainly men) who came to work at Chalk River and live in Deep River were among the best in their respective fields, and they were treated as such. Many of the original houses, the curling club, the golf course, the Catholic church and the dormitories for single staff still constitute the spine of the community.

Deep River was a new town in many ways, with a population of young parents eager and willing to get on with raising big families. My parents' neighbours each had half a dozen children, my parents five. It was a town of beginnings, and it had pretty much anything and everything a young couple might want and need to raise a family.

My parents were from New Brunswick. My father, Cyril, a teacher by training, spent his entire working life in project management for big construction companies, and the building of the Chalk River plant was the reason our family had moved to rural Ontario. His wife, Thelma (née Duffy), a nurse by training, was a stay-at-home mom. Both of my parents were devoted to family, and both strived for and achieved a middle-class life. In the truly class-divided community of Deep River, they were considered part of the professional elite and treated as such: affordable housing and relatively inexpensive medical care due to a company hospital were simply part of the perks.

My father was a touch authoritarian, liked things to go his way and was not a deeply patient man, which partly explains why he didn't work as a teacher. He would expect you to understand something immediately and to do things the way he thought they should be done, without question. He was not an unkind man, just ill-equipped to deal with the demands made on him by a time in which all the things he had been raised to believe were constantly under assault by society and his own children.

My mother raised five children and was forced to cope

with moving the family a half-dozen times to accommodate my father's work transfers. She was tough and demanding, as well as determined to please and a worrier. It was a trying combination, especially when all those different attributes were engaged at once. She would often stand in the kitchen or at the top or bottom of a set of stairs and yell, "Mary, Kathy, Peter, John or Paul . . . I don't know which one of you is doing what, but stop it now."

I was born on June 12, 1953, in Deep River, the third child and the first boy. My parents were ecstatic, and my sisters were excited as young children often are at the birth of a baby. It was by all accounts a truly joyous moment. It wouldn't be long before the joy was replaced with intensifying degrees of anxiety and worry.

Buried in the back pages of most papers that day was a report out of Geneva indicating that Canada and the United States were recording the highest number of infantile paralysis cases since the historical peak, in 1952 in Canada. Canada was seeing a 76 percent increase in infantile paralysis, and the United States a 100 percent rise. Sixty kids had come down with the disease on a military base in Whitehorse, Yukon. And the cases weren't limited to North America: the United Kingdom experienced a 50 percent increase. Those reports were just the beginning, and 1953 would turn out to be a watershed year in the polio epidemic.

2

POLIO

P olio is a devastating disease, highly infectious, easily transmitted and with no known cure. The disease attacks the spinal cord and the nervous system and, depending on the severity of the infection and the location on the spinal cord, it can paralyze muscles and tendons.

There are three basic classifications of paralytic poliomyelitis: spinal, bulbar and bulbospina, which are simply markers of the region of the central nervous system affected and the amount of inflammation and damage that result. The most common form, spinal, attacks motor neurons associated with the movement of muscles; while it can occasionally affect muscles on both sides of the body, it is usually asymmetrical. About 21 percent of all cases of paralytic polio are bulbar or bulbospina, and these cases dramatically affect the ability to breathe. When you hear polio and you think iron lung, it is patients with these forms you are picturing.

My parents and their generation were no better equipped to deal with polio than their parents or grandparents had been. Polio was first identified in 1840 and the virus isolated in early 1908, but there is clear evidence stretching back at least as far as ancient Egypt of periodic outbreaks and documented occurrences of the disease.

When I was born, contracting polio was truly a crapshoot. The disease was almost Biblical in the sense of a plague sent down by God and touching houses seemingly at random. My mother and father, like any affected parents in 1953, would have been bewildered as to why their house was targeted and not the family two doors down. Doctors weren't of much comfort, lacking any explanation for why some caught the virus and others didn't.

Much of what we now know about polio was just conjecture in the year I was born. Research has proven that polio is transmitted orally from person to person through exposure to fecal matter, which goes some way to explaining why children not yet fully toilet trained are such a prime target. Places where people gather and the virus can easily spread—swimming pools, for instance—are probable hot zones.

Polio is a disease rife with truly tricky numbers, almost inexplicable. For every thousand children under the age of five infected by the virus, only one will show any symptoms; the other 999 move about as normal, except that each is a carrier. The incubation period between infection and the appearance of symptoms is anywhere between three and thirty-five days, and everyone is most infectious in the ten-day period before symptoms can appear. The numbers are crueller for children older than six and adults, with one out of every seventy-five showing symptoms. The majority will experience what is called "abortive polio" or "non-paralytic polio," whose symptoms include "fever, sore throat, headache, vomiting, fatigue, back pain or stiffness, neck pain or stiffness, pain or stiffness in the arms or legs, muscle spasms or tenderness, and meningitis." The unlucky few, just one to three percent of those who show any symptoms at all, contract paralytic polio and experience loss of reflexes, severe muscle aches or spasms, and loose and floppy limbs, often worse on one side of the body. The onset of the actual paralysis will be sudden and is most often irreversible.

Because polio most often and most seriously affected the young, the disease was commonly referred to as "infantile paralysis." In the year I was born, little was certain about the disease other than that name, which was enough to chill the soul of even the most devout Catholic.

There is something about the word *epidemic*, especially in the context of the first half of the twentieth century, when my parents were growing up, that makes us believe there were actually five Horsemen of the Apocalypse. Cyril and Thelma were raised with a palpable fear of disease. Even in the 1950s, with declining child mortality rates, most families had experience with children dying young or being deformed for life. There were a host of diseases—chicken pox, measles, whooping cough, mumps and hepatitis—that could mark and scar your kids. Polio was simply the scariest way to lose a child to disease or leave them with a physical disability.

Polio epidemics first began appearing at the turn of the twentieth century. By 1910, much of the world—including Canada, with its first mass outbreak—was experiencing significant, startling increases in the number of cases and the severity of epidemics. As the century unfolded, epidemics came more and more frequently and lasted longer and longer. Ironically, improved sanitation, clean water and relatively efficient sewer systems created the conditions that made the epidemics possible. For much of the time polio has existed, it was ubiquitous—most people walked around having had the disease and moved on with little noticeable effect. When water supplies were made clean and sewage systems came into being, most of the population stopped being exposed to the virus, and natural exposures and immunities decreased. Communities were more vulnerable to the virus when it reappeared.

Sixty years on, it is hard to capture the sense of panic that gripped cities and towns in North America during "polio season": summer and early fall. Parents kept children indoors, public places were deserted, quarantines were put in place and victims isolated from the healthy. Every year for nearly forty years, from 1910 to 1950, an outbreak of polio took place somewhere in North America, as well as in Europe and in huge swaths of Asia and Africa.

The 1953 epidemic was the peak of a new series of infections that had begun in 1949. During those five years, 11,000 Canadians came down with polio, 9,000 in 1953 alone. Newsreels and newspapers depict a country in panic. The medical system was overwhelmed and there was a severe shortage of doctors, nurses and therapists to deal with the tsunami of cases. City and town councils argued with school officials and public health officers about whether schools should be opened and pools kept closed, and sometimes vice versa. In big cities, those who had the means fled to cottages and resorts deep in the woods, away from population centres. In a recent Discovery Channel survey of the ten worst epidemics to affect humans, polio still gets top billing, over the 1918 Spanish flu, the Black Death, HIV-AIDS and malaria.

In June 1953, the *Globe and Mail* was filled with stories about polio and possible progress in diagnosing and treating the disease. There was plenty of advice for parents on how to prevent infection: "Mak[e] sure children wash their hands often, especially after visiting the bathroom, compel all persons handling food (and this especially includes mothers) to wash their hands often, avoid small swimming pools, especially the private type in which water is not changed often, wage war on flies."

Medical practitioners and public health officials in the 1950s tried to walk an especially fine line between creating panic and instructing parents and children to act in the most responsible manner possible. In reality, the medical establishment didn't know all that much about the virus, as this *Globe and Mail* story from the time suggests:

> Although polio is the subject of one of the biggest research drives in all of medical history . . . top authorities will admit there is much they still do not know. . . . Yet all agree that parents should not become unduly alarmed: that few children are crippled of those who undergo active infection, and that far more have undergone natural immunization by mild, low grade attacks and never even knew it.

Truth be told, there wasn't much to be done anyway. There was no cure, there is still no cure, and what treatments existed in 1953 were more about alleviating symptoms than fixing the damage being done. The lack of proven treatments and of hope for a cure intensified the anxiety that all parents felt at the latest news of polio cases or pockets of polio outbreaks, and *proven* was a loaded word in itself. Treatments went in and out of fashion throughout the early twentieth century. In 1916, a typical treatment looked like this:

> Give oxygen through the lower extremities, by positive electricity. Frequent baths using almond meal, or oxidising the water. Applications of poultices of Roman chamomile, slippery elm, arnica, mustard, cantharis, amygdalae dulcis oil, and of special merit,

spikenard oil and Xanthoxolinum. Internally use
caffeine, Fl. Kola, dry muriate of quinine, elixir
of cinchone, radium water, chloride of gold, liquor
calcis and wine of pepsin.

When my parents were in their teens in the 1930s, watching friends and neighbours come down with the disease,
doctors were experimenting with hydrotherapy, elec-
trotherapy and megadoses of vitamin C. By the late 1940s
and early 1950s, when Thelma and Cyril were married and
starting a family, the conventional wisdom had changed
yet again. When I was born, physical therapies, massages,
hot and cold packs, as well as a stream of orthopaedic surgeries had been added to the arsenal of potential remedial
methods. The suggestion by medical authorities that few
children were crippled probably failed to calm most parents' frayed nerves.

Polio was big news in 1953 not just because of the outbreaks but also because of the intense race to discover a
vaccine for the disease. The quest for a vaccine had been
preoccupying the medical and scientific communities for
nearly half a century. Public health officials and governments of all stripes were keen to secure the means to
protect the general population against what was proving
to be a panic-inducing and increasingly virile plague.
Canada had a big stake in the race. Connaught Laboratories in Toronto was a major player in all aspects of the
research and had contributed significant breakthroughs

in both research and possible manufacturing processes.*

In 1953, at the height of the most damaging and widespread polio epidemic yet seen in Canada, Dr. Jonas Salk, in collaboration with Connaught Laboratories, was attempting field trials of his most promising vaccine. Mass inoculations would not start taking place in Canada until the following year, and were stopped almost immediately when a batch of contaminated vaccine actually resulted in some children contracting the disease. In Canada, the decision whether or not to continue with the vaccination programme rested with MP Paul Martin Sr., Minister of National Health and Welfare, who himself had contracted polio in 1907. His son, the future finance minister and prime minister, Paul Martin Jr., contracted the disease in 1946. Martin Sr., convinced that the standards and procedures at Canada's Connaught Labs were superior to those in the United States, ordered that the vaccinations continue. With a few remaining outbreaks of the disease, though none to match that of 1953, polio was mostly finished in Canada, though it was not until 1994 that the country was declared "polio free."

---

* It is difficult here to give this story the full weight it deserves. Many fine historians, such as Toronto-based Christopher Rutty, have worked diligently to document the history and social impact of polio, and no one tells the story of Dr. Jonas Salk and the race to create a vaccine better than Jane S. Smith in her book *Patenting the Sun: Polio and the Salk Vaccine*. In many ways the story of discovery reads like a medical thriller, though one with real consequences.

3

SEPARATED AT BIRTH

I was infected at the height of the polio season, in August 1953, just around the time Dr. Jonas Salk was performing his trials. His modern medical miracle, however, arrived too late for me. As was the norm at the time, after I fell ill, my family was quarantined. I was isolated in hospital for a year, while my parents worried and prayed at home. Isolating polio victims to stem the spread of the virus was known to be futile by 1940, but the practice continued simply to calm the public by creating a sense that something was being done.

The first signs my parents noticed—a high fever, my obvious intense discomfort and stiffness—had them panicked. All babies display a range of behaviours, but this was late summer and polio seemed to be everywhere. I turned out to be one of the lucky ones, because the damage could have been much worse. It is true that my left lower leg didn't function as such, and this would have serious ramifications over time, but at two months old at least I was alive, and I wasn't so damaged that I needed to be confined to hospital for years, as was the case with other children.

My parents were forced to stay in Deep River, my father for work, my mother to care for my siblings. I was entrusted to the medical staff at the Deep River Hospital and then at Toronto's Hospital for Sick Children for a year, with my parents visiting when they could. At the hospital, the staff first examined my stool, then took a throat swab and subjected me to a spinal tap procedure. These were the only tests available for a relatively quick diagnosis. The gold standard test involved a long needle and a tricky procedure. In the spinal tap (a lumbar puncture, to use the correct medical terminology) a needle is inserted into the lower part of the spinal cord and cerebrospinal fluid is drawn out and examined for increased white blood cells, higher-than-normal protein levels and the presence of the polio virus. If all three are present, odds are you have paralytic polio. In my case, all three were present.

The procedure is painful for adults and arguably horrific for children. The patient is positioned on his side with his knees drawn up to his chest and his back and neck straightened. The patient must be kept perfectly still, rigid even. For a number of reasons, I would undergo spinal taps at numerous points in my life, and each and every time one was ordered I experienced the closest thing I can imagine to primal dread. Even writing the words *spinal tap* causes my skin to crawl and my nerves to cringe. In some of the accounts I have read of the panic of the triage rooms in hospitals during the polio epidemics of the 1940s and '50s, the eeriest reports are those of babies and toddlers moaning as the procedure is performed. I may not remember my first lumbar puncture, but at my core is a clear, affective account of the experience.

In addition to taking the necessary diagnostic steps, the nurses fed me, tried to manage my fever and aches and pains, and, with the doctors and therapists, attempted all the latest treatment fads. This meant immobilizing my left leg, massaging the affected limb and trying to exercise the other limbs. The muscles in my left leg were paralyzed and immobilizing the limb was believed to be a way to prevent further damage and possibly give the muscles time to heal. The argument over the question of immobility versus exercise went to the very heart of medical authority. I don't know how my parents reacted to the choice of treatment options at the time, but the way they responded to later medical quandaries and dilemmas, issues I was more aware of and involved with, provided me with some clues. My mom the nurse and my dad the authoritarian were each in their own ways respectful of authority. When faced with conflicting ideas, they would have been worried, panicked and at a loss as to what was the right thing to do, before finally deciding that leaving the decision to the doctor was both the best and the wisest course of action.

As a baby, not only did I lack the means to tell nurses or doctors what or how I was feeling, but it wouldn't always have been clear how I was responding to the various types of treatments and exercises I was being given. Fixing my limbs and moving my limbs would have involved a lot of guesswork

and day-to-day adjustments. As a growing baby, my development was soon completely out of whack. At a point when you
might expect spontaneous turning and rolling and crawling,
I was doing none of that, and no one was quite sure when,
how or if I might start.

I can never be certain how much of my time as an infant
being treated in hospital for polio was centred on the Kenny
Method, named for a world-famous Australian nurse, Sister
Elizabeth Kenny. During the 1930s she rebelled against
the conventional wisdom of immobilizing, insisting that
the best treatment for polio was heat wraps and active and
passive exercising of the affected limbs and muscles. It is
clear from contemporaneous documents that, as much as
possible, nurses and physiotherapists were intent on finding ways to get bodies and limbs moving, and where that
wasn't possible, they put in place the aids and tools necessary to help those who had been paralyzed by polio to adapt.

In my case, at the age of fourteen months, that meant
some tendon surgery, where damaged tendons are supple-
mented by the transfer of healthy ones to weaker areas in
the body. You can still see a small scar that travels down the
inside of my left leg where an attempt was made to try to
repair and/or supplement the tendons that worked to raise
and lower my foot. It didn't work, but it is my understanding that it was a faint hope anyway. The doctors, the nurses
and my parents all understood that walking was going to be
a problem, but they decided to give every option a go before
sending me home. As a consequence of the tendon surgery,

and in an effort to provide some stability to a baby who had truly limited use of one leg, the doctors put my left leg in a cast, an early version of what we now call a walking cast. The nurses and doctors knew that, once we were home, my learning to walk was going to be a family undertaking. My parents would supply the patience and guidance while I, not yet a year and a half old, would have to supply the stubbornness.

4

BABY STEPS

In Deep River, all the houses on our street were crowded with newborns, toddlers, small children and preteens. This new town filled with young scientists and their wives had inadvertently created a living laboratory for raising children. There were opportunities to share joys and disappointments, to touch base with others going through just what you were trying to cope with, and there were places to go for reassurance, tips, warnings. New parents at that time may not have had social media, but they did have stay-at-home mothers, extended families and the burgeoning self-help sub-genre of "bringing up baby." It was an age when advances in the keeping of medical records, in data collection and collation, and in the development of standards and benchmarks in all areas of life was the new norm.

My parents wanted normal kids (what parents don't?) and I was a real challenge to that whole idea. By the time I came home from the hospital, there were two more children in the house. My mother had given birth to twin boys while I was hospitalized and now we were a family of seven. One of my sisters later told me that when my father and mother were setting off to get me from the hospital, she insisted they leave me there because the house had too many children already. In that small house in Deep River, in addition to my parents and an uncle who was living with us, there were five children between the ages of two months and eight years. 110 Algonquin Street was already a chaotic family home; the fact that I had real development issues complicated everything immensely.

What made all of this even more difficult for my parents, and for my siblings and me, was that we moved a lot. In the first fifteen years of my life, I lived in seven provinces. Learning to walk was a process I tackled first in Deep River and then in Buckingham, Quebec, where my father was involved in the construction of a pulp and paper plant. My father's work meant that we hung around in a community only until a project was finished, and then we moved on to the next big project that the construction company was beginning. No sooner had my mother and father settled in, grown accustomed to the community, created friends and networks of support, found schools, doctors and in my case specialists, than they would have to pack up and move yet again.

As a curious six-year-old, I discovered in my parents' bookcase a well-thumbed volume that had clearly been in the household for years. It was that classic of the parenting self-help movement, first published in 1946, *The Common Sense Book of Baby and Child Care* by Benjamin Spock. It was the most popular reference guide to that universal but very individual question, "My baby is x months old—what should he be doing now?" Some of the answers, for various stages in the baby's development, involved mobility—from crawling to walking.

We have goals for how humans develop. These are the underpinning of all pediatric medicine and all parental anxiety. My parents were no different from parents of any time, filled with doubt and worry. The only constant is that each generation creates and receives its own methods for dealing with the issues that arise. Regardless of what polio might mean to the rest of my life, when I returned home from the hospital the big issue, the key questions, centred on how and when I would learn to walk.

Learning to walk as a baby is the subject of much conjecture, research and analysis. Despite the fact that, in evolutionary terms, human beings have been walking since before we were humans, much of what we know is an odd mix of guesswork, tentative fact and understanding. Walking begins when a baby pulls himself upright to the point where he can take steps on his own, unaided. Before that there is rolling over, lifting the chest, flexing the legs and arms, crawling. The estimates of how much time a toddler puts into learning to walk range from 1,000 hours to 10,000 hours. Some analysts suggest that the average baby spends as much time learning to walk as an Olympic athlete does preparing for the Games. If we crunch these numbers, 1,000 hours, even at eight hours a day, works out to be 125 days, or a little over four full months. And 10,000 hours works out to 1,250 eight-hour days, or forty-one months, or three and a half years of effort, concentration and time. The researchers will tell you the 1,000-hour estimate is the amount of time necessary for secure and steady walking, while the 10,000 hours reflects the full process of fixing one's "normal gait," which is not completed until some point in one's teen years.

Despite any and every attempt to map and plot out how children develop any skill or ability, what every expert acknowledges is that each child is different. One fairly standard parental guide on gross motor development and learning to walk during the first three years breaks down the stages of the process while stressing that "variation is common":

> **6 weeks:** sits with curved back, needs support. Head control developing.
>
> **4 months:** no head lag.
>
> **6–7 months:** sits with self-propping (hands pushing down on legs as he sits). Stands with support.
>
> **9 months:** gets into sitting position alone.
>
> **10 months:** pulls to standing and stands holding on.
>
> **12 months:** stands and walks with one hand held.
>
> **15 months:** walks independently (broad-based, high stepping), stoops to pick up objects. Creeps up stairs.

18 months: climbs stairs holding rail. Runs. More mature gait when walking. Seats self in chair.

21 months: walks backwards with imitation. Walks upstairs, two feet per step.

2 years: goes up and down stairs alone.

2½ years: jumps with both feet. Walks on tiptoe when asked.

3 years: able to stand on one foot for a few seconds.

In one sense, there is no arguing with this guide. Eagerly awaited milestones are what they are, and missing them creates stress for parents and relatives. Children are largely unaware that they have missed the moment, though the lack of independence that not being able to walk entails does chafe. Being a child is a job just like any other, and there are things children need to do even when they can't articulate what it is they haven't accomplished. Children can pick up on hidden and not so hidden signals from a parent that perhaps they are not living up to expectations, not progressing as quickly as a sibling or the younger child next door. While the motor milestone as the "hallmark of young children's emerging independence" is without doubt true, it was not the case with most infants suffering from paralytic polio, including myself.

When I finally came home from the hospital, I was about fifteen months old but really at the nine- to ten-month stage, when I was just learning to get into a sitting position and pull myself up. Apparently I never mastered crawling, but considering the circumstances, that makes some sense: I was doing all this catch-up while wearing a plaster cast on my leg.

Casts, both short (lower part of the leg) and long (full leg), were used to help prevent the weakened and floppy limb from becoming twisted and bent out of shape. They also provided much-needed stability for an infant whose muscles and nerves were insufficiently developed to allow for any of the natural emergent activities involved in turning any and all of us into walkers. So the cast gave me something to stand on, and a place to push off from. The cast made possible those two phases of walking: stance and swing.

It is a good thing I had the cast, because my parents weren't sure how to teach me to walk. It wasn't their fault; most of us would be at a loss trying to explain to an infant how to progress from crawling to walking. I don't have clear memories of learning to walk that first time, but I have been told that I was a remarkably stubborn infant, which doesn't surprise friends who know me as an adult. Apparently, after learning to haul myself up to a standing position, I proceeded to stumble and hitch and haltingly walk around the house.

My mother, who never talked with much if any laughter about my growing up, did once tell me that I was from time to time annoyingly insistent about trying to go everywhere possible in the house. She had to keep an eye out for me while dealing with the needs and demands of four other children. The washing machine was in the basement of our house and one time when my mother went downstairs to do laundry, I followed. Navigating stairs was something I had not yet accomplished, and I launched myself off the top step into the air, plummeted down into the basement and landed straight up on my cast, somewhat surprised but unhurt. She told me that story with a bit of a chuckle and added that I hadn't seemed frightened by the event, and in fact was laughing as I stood looking around at the basement, a part of the house I had not yet discovered.

In reading about polio treatment styles and techniques in the developing world, I was fascinated to discover that some children in India and Africa who are stricken with polio as infants never learn to walk but spend their lives crawling, or the equivalent of crawling. There is so much associated with walking beyond the idea of locomotion and mobility. Walking can denote status, attitude and psychological state. Look at teen boys, fashion models, athletes or even criminals and police officers: walking speaks volumes. Not walking speaks more quietly but just as powerfully. Doctors who intervene in later life with surgical remedies can often create the situation where the adult learns to walk as the child never could. To imagine a life spent crawling and then finally learning to walk, and how an individual would process all of that, sometimes leaves me lost in wonder.

You know how some parents bronze the first pair of baby shoes? It's a memento of a historic moment, a milestone in their child's life. My parents would have had to bronze a plaster cast, as arguably my first shoe was a walking cast. My second shoe opened up a whole new world of possibility, and of difficulty.

5

THE CRIPPLE

Getting to the point where I could walk was pretty much a solo effort, as it is with other children. Parents encourage and enthuse, but learning to flex muscles, stand, negotiate balance, move, sequence and move again are barriers that one has to conquer oneself. Once I got to the stage where I could walk, it didn't take me all that long to realize that walking for me was different than it was for just about anyone I knew, certainly different from everyone else in my family. Walking for me was hard, awkward and painful. And if others didn't at first notice my awkward stance and swing, the brace and the shoes gave it all away.

I learned early on that just because you hate something doesn't mean it will go away or be fixed. I hated that brace. I hated my shoes almost from my first awareness of them. I got my first brace around my second birthday, after I had learned to walk, in a fashion, with the aid of the cast. A very early memory is the feeling of constriction around my left leg, especially the lower part of the leg. I have always sensed my two legs differently, even as a child, perhaps especially as a child. One leg moved freely, one needed support. One leg felt free, one felt confined. The difference was the brace and the shoes.

First the brace. It was made of two steel bars that ran up the sides of my left leg, from the heel to just below the knee. The ends of the bars were inserted into the built-up heel of the shoe. Just below the knee, the bars slid into slots in a leather strap that ran around the leg and was fastened with a buckle to keep everything in place. The brace seemed heavy, it was heavy, and I was constantly aware of its presence. How could I not be? I wore this brace twenty-four hours a day, seven days a week. The one exception was when I was having a bath. I wore the brace and shoe to bed, slept in them. Naturally, the heavy shoe and the brace tended to tear at sheets. My mother's solution was to cover the brace and shoe with oversized heavy socks. Getting into bed was a process.

As a child, even before going to school, before understanding the idea of a mind-body identity problem, I knew a fundamental truth: I was the brace and the brace was me. What perplexed and angered me was that even with the brace and the shoes, my walking was far from normal, involving a serious limp and a hitch in my gait, the result of one leg being shorter, frailer and weaker than the other. To my six-year-old self, my walk was just another piece of evidence that life was unfair.

The shoes were actually part of the brace, and vice versa.

No ordinary shoes could accommodate the built-up heel and sole necessary for my shorter leg and the brace. So where other children had lightweight runners for school or oxfords for church, I got clunky black orthopaedic shoes. Even though as a three-year-old I had as little fashion sense as I do as a sixty-year-old, I knew that "special" shoes make you stand out. If wrestling with the brace wasn't sufficiently distressing, the brace and the shoes were a killer combination. The shoes had to be different sizes because my feet were different sizes, with the paralyzed leg significantly smaller. My parents had to buy two different-sized pairs of shoes and use the left from the smaller pair and the right from the larger pair.

Naturally, none of this was cheap. This was the 1950s, before the creation of the national health care system and before workplace health insurance. My parents had to shell out for shoes and braces on a regular basis, given that both the braces and the shoes needed to be replaced as I grew. Luckily for my parents, the folks who made orthopaedic shoes charged for only a pair and a half instead of the two pairs I actually needed.

There were additional costs associated with my needs: new sheets to replace the ones I wore out, creams and ointments to soothe the chafing caused by the brace and heavy shoes, plus the expenses you never imagine. I remember, with the vividness that deeply embarrassing moments create, a new chesterfield that quickly developed tears from my sitting on it wearing my shoes, as of course I had to do. My parents complained to the store that the quality of the sofa was inferior, but the store insisted the material was fine and that my parents should just keep me off the couch if I had to wear shoes. I remember the angry encounter between my parents and the sales clerk with a clarity that doesn't accompany my other memories as a six-year-old.

The shoes, and by extension me, were also the object of derision, stares and insults by other children. Boys and girls would point and stare, I'd be given nasty nicknames, and jokes would be made about my status as a cripple. In those days, this type of name-calling and ridicule were largely written off as "boys will be boys." I remember parents whispering to children who were fascinated or repelled by my limp or my brace that "it wasn't polite to stare" and I realized that of course I was someone to be stared at. As a child, and even today as an adult, I believed that the shoes were the magnet for the attention that made me a target.

So it will probably come as no real surprise that shoes have always mattered to me, probably more than any other item of clothing.

I grew up in a family of five children, all of whom, except for me, wore sneakers. When you sleep wearing a rigid device that weighs two pounds and rips sheets, you dream of running in sneakers. I had those dreams for years. I still do.

When I was six and off to school, my doctors concluded that I could spend a small amount of time each week not wearing my brace. In other words, I could wear sneakers,

I could be like every other kid, even if only for a few hours on a Saturday.

I remember the first time I wore sneakers. We were living in Saint-Eustache, Quebec, a small town on the outskirts of Montreal. My parents had moved us there when my father went to work on the construction of Place Ville Marie in Montreal. We had the upper floor of a duplex, with long metal stairs in the back leading to a huge central field where the neighbourhood kids played. Those stairs were awkward to climb and descend, and my heavy shoes would clang on each step. On this very special Saturday, a sunny spring morning, I put on my sneakers for the very first time and raced, as only a child who has never raced and never learned to run can, down the back stairs into the field looking for my friends.

Childhood friends were never my strong suit. I spent a lot of time in hospitals, I wore a brace, I limped, and even as a kid I was pretty cerebral. And of course we moved frequently, and every time we did, it meant having to create new friendships. So friends were pretty much a neighbourhood thing, based on proximity rather than interests. We hung out because we lived next door to each other. I was the cripple who lived down the street.

This morning I was on edge, vibrating with excitement. Those sneakers felt just as I'd imagined they would: light, barely there. I was flying even before I put my foot to the ground.

I ran down the pathways separating the backyards of the neighbourhood to catch up with the other children. But those whom I'd thought were my friends jeered at me, pelted me with fruit and other stuff lying in the weeds on the edges of yards, and ran off, as only kids who have spent years learning to run can. I was left trying to integrate and internalize whether their actions were those of bullies intent on beating me down or an act of respect indicating that the cripple could now be treated just like any other kid because he wore sneakers. Trying to make sense of bullying was nothing new to me.

Ultimately, though, it didn't matter because this day was really about the sneakers. Sneakers became a badge of normalcy, an indicator of sameness. My relationship with sneakers is lifelong and complicated, and I may be somewhat more sophisticated and aware now than I was as a six-year-old, but it is still true that when I see sneakers, I see freedom. Then and now, sneakers were about magical thinking, and they weren't the only such totems in my life.

6

FAITH HEALING

My parents, both Irish Canadians, were deeply devout Catholics. This meant Mass at least once a week, a daily saying of the rosary by the whole family, a near-abject obedience to the musings, wishes and orders that flowed from Rome and whatever diocese we found ourselves in after each move, meatless Fridays, days of obligation, nightly prayers, Sunday school and, where possible, a Catholic school for the children. Catholicism was the guide to living, the answer to life's difficulties, the promise of salvation, and the source of comfort and of explanations when things went wrong or bad things happened to good, or at least innocent, people.

The religion my parents passed on, the religion my deeply pious grandparents ensured was learned, absorbed and regurgitated by their children and especially their grandchildren on every visit through church services, large family prayers and a constant discussion of God, sin and Church, was a pre–Vatican II Catholicism immersed in incense, Latin, foreboding, structure and stricture. It was a demanding faith and it was a relatively simple faith. All one had to do was follow the rules, be true and await one's reward. When things went wrong, my parents' Catholicism was comforting and ultimately a haven.

My siblings and I grew up with the truth that God worked in mysterious ways, that God never gave you a burden too great to shoulder or a cross too heavy to bear. We were taught to never complain about our trials, tribulations or sorrows. We were taught that God had a plan and that there was a reward for accepting God's plan and doing God's will. We also learned that children were special, like lambs unto the Lord, and that parents were held responsible for their own sins and the sins of their offspring.

Religion was a true solace for my parents, but it was also a source of guilt and worry. They had taken to heart the idea that injury or harm to a child might flow from the misdeeds or lapses of the parents. Their prayers for intercession were constant, as constant as our nightly sessions of saying the rosary. Whatever physical problems I was experiencing were a form of testing, a trial. Life's pains and tribulations were simply a way station on the path to life everlasting. As a consequence, for all of my life, how I have understood walking and the problems I have with walking have never been far from odd traces and strands of religious dogma.

Unintentionally, or so I have to believe, one of the lessons I was made to absorb from this atmosphere of religious fervour and thinking was my parents' and the Church's sense of guilt—for the angst and anguish I was inflicting on others through my physical problems and the demands made by the reality of my physical deformities. At six, the guilt was at least inchoate; I just somehow knew that I had inadvertently changed the lives of my two older sisters and my two younger brothers.

I also desperately wanted to be normal and fit in with everyone else, and I was never certain why I couldn't. Faith-based explanations never truly cut it with me, though I do remember what seemed at the time to be intensely valiant efforts to accept that having polio, experiencing difficulties walking, and standing out from the crowd were somehow part of God's plan and as such were to be accepted and even celebrated. I was taught to pray, at home and in church, offering up my suffering for the good of others, reciting set formulas acknowledging the pain endured by Christ and his early followers. The power of prayer and the lessons of others were things I believed in, things I hoped would make me more accepting of who I was.

Of course, none of this meant that I, or my parents, couldn't pray for some form of miracle, some unexpected development that might make me whole and sound. Catholics believe in that type of divine intervention. Every time we said a rosary as a family, we offered up special pleas for a sick family member, a troubled neighbour. At every Mass, special interventions were sought for a troubled member of the parish. After all, Lourdes, with all its excesses and its more than five million pilgrims a year, exists solely because of the belief on the part of devout and desperate Catholics that sufficient piety, sufficient faith can move mountains and change medical realities.

And not just Lourdes. After all, we lived in Montreal, home to St. Joseph's Oratory, centrepiece of the story of Brother André, as of 2010 called Saint Brother André or Saint André. André Bessette spent his life as a lay brother with the Congregation of the Holy Cross in Montreal. He often cared for the sick and the lame, and was a keen devotee of Saint Joseph and a believer in the ability of the saints to heal. Saint André was a powerful figure in the history of Quebec, and his death in 1937 was a moment of national mourning, with more than a million people attending the visitation before his burial. He was a truly mythic and compelling figure for Catholics, especially Catholics in need of a miracle. Thousands have credited Saint André with cures of the most debilitating of illnesses.

My mother and father truly believed that seeking the intercession of Saint André and Saint Joseph could provoke miraculous healing, so we prayed and visited the Oratory both when we lived in Montreal and later, on visits to the city. The Basilica of St. Joseph's Oratory began as a small chapel and is now a national shrine and the largest church in Canada. When you go to the Basilica, whether as one of the two million who make the pilgrimage each year or out of simple curiosity, you approach the building by climbing 283 stone steps. The truly devout climb 99 of those steps on their knees, something my mother did but I didn't. Seeking a saintly intervention is not for the weak of will. When you finally reach the inner sanctum, you are faced with the image, power and meaning of the thousands of crutches, made of wood, metal and plastic, abandoned by the healed and covering the walls.

The Bible, both the Old and New Testaments, is filled with references to cripples and the lame, and there are many unfortunate equations of sin, forgiveness, the lame and healing. Matthew 9 is but one example:

> Jesus stepped into a boat, crossed over and came to his own town. Some men brought to him a paralyzed man, lying on a mat. When Jesus saw their faith, he said to the man, "Take heart, son; your sins are forgiven." At this, some of the teachers of the law said to themselves, "This fellow is blaspheming!" Knowing their thoughts, Jesus said, "Why do you entertain evil thoughts in your hearts? Which is easier: to say, 'Your sins are forgiven,' or to say, 'Get up and walk'? But I want you to know that the Son of Man has authority on earth to forgive sins." So he said to the paralyzed man, "Get up, take your mat and go home." Then the man got up and went home. When the crowd saw this, they were filled with awe; and they praised God, who had given such authority to man.

This seeking of a miracle, this beseeching of the Lord, is a delicate dance. It needed an approach that was more slant than direct. The prayer to Saint André was and is a masterpiece of coded supplication:

Brother André,

We celebrate your presence among us. Your loving
friendship with Jesus, Mary and Joseph makes
you a powerful intercessor with God, our Father.
Compassion carries your words straight to God's
heart, and your prayers are answered and bring
comfort and healing. Through you, from our lips to
God's ear, our supplications are heard. . . . We ask
to be made a part of God's work, alongside you, in
the spirit of prayer, compassion and humility.
Brother André, pray for us. Amen.

My parents and extended family weren't, given the time
and their faith, off the wall with their thoughts about God's
healing power. They believed and still believe in miracles,
the power of prayer and the value of pure intentions and
pure hearts. At the same time, they did not eschew the
world of medicine and science. They took me and my siblings to doctors when needed. They filled prescriptions,
took drugs and listened to doctors without blinking an
eye. My parents saw themselves as modern, believers in
both the wonders of science and the power of God. They
did not recognize any contradiction in the simultaneous
holding of these two sets of beliefs and understandings.
The possibility of faith healing was a constant, but in the
meantime, investigating the options offered by doctors
was equally necessary.

I think this attempt to balance the miraculous and the scientific must have been hardest on my mother. The most common description one hears about her from any and all of my relatives: Thelma was a saint. Sometimes sainthood is thrust upon a person.

In the 1950s and 1960s, when a child was ill, care of the child fell on the mother. That burden was clearly at the heart of a truly traumatic event experienced by some of my siblings and myself when we were living in Saint-Eustache when I was six. We had gone as a pack, mother and four children, to the store around the corner from where we lived. While in the store, my mother became agitated and insisted we go home immediately, shooing us outside and onto the sidewalk. Suddenly she collapsed to the ground, shaking, in a seizure-like state. My siblings and I became hysterical, screaming—in English in this largely French community— for someone to call an ambulance.

The next thing I remember is being in the kitchen of our house, my parents' friends and my dad explaining to us that our mother was in the hospital getting care for nervous exhaustion. I remember hearing that she was getting a drug, phenobarbital, that was going to help make her better. But we were also told that we had to "behave," be less of a bother and somehow be better kids so that our mom would get better. This lecture, this insistence that we correct our unspecified behaviours, would become a constant refrain over the years.

The emotions I experienced then, and have continued to experience throughout my life, ranged from shame to guilt, with a significant stop at fear. I was learning—and it was a lesson that would be repeated—that my behaviour, my demands, my health would be and were, in combination with those of my siblings, the critical factors in our mother's state of health. I was too young then to feel the anger that naturally arises when in effect you are being blamed for the poor health of another. That anger came when I was in my late teens and twenties, and no longer inclined to accept responsibility for my mother's condition. Using guilt to change children's behaviour is a classic parental move, and while I have tried desperately to avoid doing any such thing as a parent myself, I have to imagine that I have done so either intentionally or unintentionally, blatantly or subtly.

It was around this time, during my mother's first bout of intense illness, that I had the first of a series of conversations with my father about planning for my life. We talked a lot about my going into some job or career that would take into account and be accommodating of my disability and my problems with walking. I was six. To this day I remember being advised by him that I should consider becoming a pharmacist and having my own pharmacy. I suspect it was well-meaning advice that simply emerged from his sense of what types of roles might be open to a person with a clear and likely permanent problem. It was outside his experience to suggest that I might make my living with my writing, and when that began to happen he seemed pleased, but I have always suspected he may still have wanted me to be a pharmacist.

My mother returned from the hospital for all intents and purposes in decent health, and I am not sure how long she needed anticonvulsants and sedatives, but we were all reassured that things were getting back to normal. In our case, especially as far as I was concerned, it was a faint and ultimately false hope.

7

THE EXPERIMENT

We moved to Calgary, Alberta, from Saint-Eustache, Quebec, when I was eight years old. The construction company my father worked for had a number of contracts and projects under way with the Distant Early Warning network being built by the Canadian and American governments in the northern reaches of Canada. Calgary was where my father's part of the operation was based.

Calgary was a city of 270,000 people in 1961. The economy was pretty much oil, gas, farming and ranching. We thought of it as a big city and we lived in the northwest quadrant in a salmon-pink ranch-style bungalow with a chain-link-fenced backyard. All of us kids went to the local Catholic school.

My memories of Calgary are naturally fragmentary, but one set of recollections is very clear: those associated with a medical experiment intended to make it easier for me to walk.

Alberta was one of the areas of Canada that had been hit hard by the polio epidemic of 1953, and the province's entire history with the disease had led to big changes in the practice of medicine, the funding of medical research and the treatment of polio victims. On average every year during the "fall epidemic" polio season, the disease accounted for one-quarter to one-third of all admissions at the Children's Hospital in Calgary. As early as 1937, with the passage of the Poliomyelitis Sufferers Act, the province began taking all the steps it could to combat the virus, including throwing money at the problem. By 1959, the per-patient day fee paid by the province to the Calgary Children's Hospital for polio patients was $10.25; for other orthopaedic patients it was $3.40. The combination of money and the sheer volume of stricken kids put the province at the forefront of the nation's fight against the disease. Other key initiatives included the restructuring of orthopaedic surgery departments and the emphasis that medical schools put on researching remedial measures to be used with polio victims. Doctors in the province were famous throughout Canada and the United States for experimentation, especially when it came to polio victims. It was literally a wild west for medical experiments to correct or eliminate the damage done by the disease.

My main problem, the mismatch in the lengths of my legs, was by no means an unusual one. Iron lungs may be the iconic image of the era of polio epidemics, but shrivelled, weak, deformed or misshapen limbs were the norm, so common that if you meet a person of a certain age and they limp or have a weakened arm, odds are they experienced paralytic polio at some point.

Finding the ways and means to match leg length is simple in theory and remarkably difficult in practice, and that was especially true in the early 1960s, when doctors everywhere, including Calgary, were faced with hundreds of cases of varying degrees of urgency. At the time, there were two schools of thought, two common approaches: you could find the means to stop or impede the growth of the longer leg and thereby allow the smaller leg to catch up, or you could try to lengthen the shorter leg through different forms of surgery.

When I arrived in Calgary and was taken by my parents to the hospital for yet another consultation with yet another set of doctors, it was just in time to be enlisted in a medical experiment. My doctors wanted to open up a third possible avenue of remedial medicine. They were eager to see if you could accelerate the growth rate of the smaller limb so that it would grow faster and in time catch up with the unaffected leg. When I write that sentence today, I have several reactions. Firstly, I shake my head at the thought of just how complicated the whole idea is. Secondly, I have to wonder what went through my parents' minds as they considered the idea. Thirdly, I am truly at a loss as to how I would react today if a doctor made such a suggestion to me about either my child or myself. What would I do or say?

I know from later conversations with my mother that one of the things my parents did was consult their parish priest and explain to him how concerned they were. It was an experimental procedure, they wanted the best for me, they wanted if possible to make me better or more whole, and they hoped they might be able to move us all past the lingering effects of the polio. But they were scared. They didn't know what to do. Their priest told them to trust in God, and by that he simply meant: listen to the doctors. It was a suggestion that by nature they were prone to accept.

My parents, like most of their generation, were obsequious when it came to medical opinion. What a doctor said, believed, suggested was good enough for them. And in many situations, that type of adherence to conventional wisdom makes a great deal of sense. But it's one thing when your doctor is prescribing an antibiotic or suggesting a change in your diet; it's quite another if they are suggesting a radical and untried surgical procedure.

The thinking of the doctors as I reconstruct it—what with records being remarkably scarce and published papers on experimental orthopaedic techniques not the norm in the late 1950s and 1960s—goes as follows: There are tumours that sometimes occur in limbs that result in increased blood flow to the affected limb. One of the consequences of the tumour and the increased blood flow can be an accelerated growth of the limb. So what if you could mimic the effects of the tumour without the tumour being present? What if the blood flow in the shortened leg could be increased such that the limb grew faster than the normal-length leg? Would the result be, in time, legs of equal length? Given the prevailing attitudes and the "think outside the box" culture of orthopaedic surgery in Alberta at the time, this was just the type of idea that excited everyone on the medical side.

On the patient and family side, if this wild theory might actually work, it was seemingly the best chance that I could be made normal.

Standards of medical behaviour evolve, and ideas about consent, informed consent and proportionality of problem versus proposed solution are much different in 2014 than they were in 1961. At a time and in a place where the ravages of the polio epidemic were constantly on display, finding remedies was a high priority for patients, parents and doctors. According to numerous memoirs of Alberta doctors who grappled with polio, they weren't simply driven by the institutional resources made available for polio treatments as opposed to other forms of care, though the accounts clearly indicate that was one factor at play. With thousands of young people around North America trying to cope with the consequences of paralysis and mangled or stunted limbs, the pressure to find a range of possible solutions was intense. All of the perceived wisdom, knowledge and technique lay with the doctors. Every parent was expected to be willing to try anything that might help their child, and the victims themselves were encouraged and expected to be willing and excited about any and every possibility. As one history of surgery in Alberta puts it, "For physicians who were on the front lines polio was the absolute basis for all learning. Surgeons around the world used polio epidemics to experiment with new techniques, especially once the advent of antibiotics removed the fear of infecting joints during surgery, and their developments soon came to be used internationally."

In the end, my parents agreed to this experimental and very rare surgery and I was admitted to hospital. I was nine, but hospitals are scary places regardless of how old you are. Over time I would grow very familiar, way too intimate, with the routines and protocols of hospital life. You are surrounded by strangers who take control of everything; your family are simply visitors who check in on you from time to time. Basic issues such as what and when to eat, when to sleep, and the structure of your day all become part and parcel of the agenda and routines of folks dressed largely in white—or at least that's how I saw it at the time and remember it to this day. But despite my growing familiarity with the situation, I never came to cope well with the scary part. I worried all the time I was in hospital, and I was very lonely. My parents saw me as much as possible, but visits by children were frowned upon, so I didn't see my siblings. My parents' visits were never extended affairs, as my dad had his job and my mother had four other children to raise. So I spent a lot of time alone, reading, enduring frequent physical examinations, and trying to fathom those conversations adults have about you while acting as if you aren't even in the room.

The evening prep before surgery was difficult. Strangers appeared and washed my body with antiseptic soap, administered an enema, stopped serving me food and water, and then told me to go to sleep and that they would take me to surgery the next morning. It goes without saying that I didn't sleep well or much. A real disadvantage of an active imagination is that your nightmare scenarios occur while you are wide awake.

But the morning of surgery was even worse. Someone I'd never met before came to get me very early, took me from my room, put me on a strange bed in a room full of other people I had never met, all waiting for their own operations. All the staff were walking around with masks on and I couldn't really figure out what was happening, when it was going to happen, or even why. New strangers came and gave me needles, hooked up machines, spread iodine-like swatches across my stomach, groin and leg. I was almost at the point of bursting into great sobs of fear when yet another person wearing a mask came and wheeled my bed out of the room and down a corridor, and I was moving fast and my eyes were going every which way trying to figure out *what now?* Then my bed was pushed through big swinging doors and I was in a large room filled with people in gowns, masks and gloves and a couple grabbed me and lifted me up onto a big cold metal table, and while one of these masked people was sliding needles into one of my arms, a second was wrapping a blood pressure gauge around another arm, and a third person, who was actually behind me and whom I couldn't see, slid a mask over my face and the air started to taste funny and a voice asked me to count backwards from 100 and I did . . . 100 . . . 99 . . . 98 . . . and before I got very far, the world vanished.

During this surgery, a long incision was made in the upper inside portion of my left thigh, and through the fusing of some of the major arteries and veins of the leg, everything was in essence rewired, forcing an increased blood flow to the leg. The surgery was complicated and lasted nearly five hours. The next thing I knew, I was slowly becoming aware of things: I could see a clock, I knew I was in a bed with metal sides, I was hooked up to a machine and very thirsty and feeling very weak. When I looked down, my left leg was wrapped in thick bandages and I hurt everywhere and was so, so sleepy.

I spent the next few weeks in the hospital recovering from the surgery and becoming reacquainted with how to walk. By this point, the hospital was slightly less scary but no less lonely. I was experiencing a slight, strange sense of disappointment. I didn't actually feel much different and it seemed to me that, given all the drama, I should have felt something, but I didn't. All I felt was lonely and slightly bored as I did physio, learned how to care for my incision and regained a bit of the physical strength that major surgery always robs a person of. Once I had accomplished those post-operative necessities, with the incision healed, I was discharged. I was instructed simply to go about as I had been up until then, though my parents and I were told that in about three years' time I would need surgery to undo the leg rewiring, regardless of whether or not the experiment had succeeded.

8

MY SIBLINGS,
MY DISABILITY AND ME

Tolstoy writes in *Anna Karenina*, "Happy families are all alike; every unhappy family is unhappy in its own way," and our family was much more the unhappy family than the happy one.

I've always felt separate from my family; in fact, some of my earliest memories are of a distance between them and me. It is not that my brothers and sisters and I don't love each other or aren't somewhat fond of one another, but there has always been a sense that the connections are fragile and tenuous. There were significant moments growing up when my absence from them or their absence from me was real in both a time-space continuum sense and a psycho-spiritual sense.

It was perfectly understandable, even if hurtful. My sisters are older, and were engaged in forging a family life all of their own before the pesky, sickly brother came along. My brothers, twins and younger, were born when I was in hospital and actually spent the first months of their lives unaware of my existence. In addition, the girls (being girls) had their own particular issues and perspectives to work out, and the brothers (being twins) had their intimate bond that created its own dynamic while also affecting everyone else in the house.

There is also the normal reality that children, even siblings, aren't as empathetic or sympathetic to the troubles of others as we might like or even need. I didn't walk right, couldn't really run, wasn't always up for physical games, never learned to ride a bicycle and was an outsider at some very basic level. From my perspective, I was like Rudolph waiting for a foggy Christmas Eve that never comes. From their perspective—who knows?

Over the years, I have looked at a fair amount of literature on birth order and the immediate and lingering effects a disabled sibling has on family dynamics, and the reality is generally not pretty. One of my sisters recently summed it up when she wrote me, offering advice for this book and suggesting I just be honest and express how from time to time my siblings were shits. They would and did complain about the "special" treatment and attention I seemed to need and sometimes demanded. Their resentment could take the form of shoving and other physical lashing out, or isolation and a form of sibling shunning. Often it boiled down to the distinction between them and me: they were a cohesive unit and I was the outsider, the one who was absent from time to time.

Without doubt, this dynamic played out in reverse as well. Kids with chronic health problems aren't saints and are capable of doing wrong, being selfish or attempting to arrange matters in the way that suits them best. I could be and was at times mean, cranky, whiny, judgmental and capable of pleading for special treatment because I was the sick kid—demanding to sit in the front seat of a car jammed with five children and two adults, insisting on the attention I craved regardless of the problems my sisters and brothers, not to mention our parents, might be dealing with.

I was a childhood bully, using my intellect and sharp tongue, even at an early age, in place of the size and agility other bullies possessed. I remember being in grade one, religious studies. We had been assigned a section of the New Testament as homework the day before and our teacher was reviewing the lesson. She asked a boy sitting next to me how Joseph, Mary and the baby Jesus had made it to Egypt from Bethlehem while fleeing Herod's troops. My six-year-old classmate, a boy who either hadn't done his homework, hadn't absorbed it or was confused by the question, replied, "By train?" I just laughed out loud, raucously. Then I hooted, "'By train'—that is the dumbest thing I have ever heard. By train?! They took a donkey." Of course I was made to go sit in the corner and reflect on my behaviour, but I still remember thinking, *Whoa, that is dumb*. As I said, kids with health problems aren't saints. I have always had a decent mind, a good memory and a great vocabulary, and I have used these attributes with wicked cruelty more times than I can count. No one was better at finding the apt word, the precise adjective that, used as a weapon, could make another child cry.

I believe that this ability and inclination to bully was a

response to the teasing and bullying I myself received at school, a defence mechanism that allowed me to feel better about myself in the face of others' ridicule. Though my siblings sometimes hit or scorned me, they also looked out for me. One of my sisters told me that she remembers coming home from school and asking my mother what a gimp was "because a boy at school called Peter that." She told me that our mother burst into tears and told her it was an ignorant, cruel word. The next day my sister got in trouble with the principal because she hit the name caller and told him that he couldn't call a person a gimp.

My brothers were typical boys, fond of fooling around and being quite physical, and that wasn't my speed, ever. So on numerous occasions, what they might have regarded as fun—stealing a crutch, punching my leg or hip, tripping me as I walked by—was seen and experienced by me in a much different light. I felt put upon, like their target. We couldn't always work this out between us, largely because they ended up being yelled at or punished by my parents. I was frustrated by these interventions, which my brothers saw as special treatment for me and unfair treatment for them, largely because I was trying to figure out if I was as sensitive or fragile as my parents thought and partly because, however fragile I might be, I didn't really want to be that person who needed constant protection.

I was not averse to getting my own back when and where I could. I was great at insults and verbal gymnastics and I have a very caustic wit. I could and did make my sisters cry, could and did enrage my brothers with my words, provoking them into a physical response for which I knew they would be punished. I could and did enjoy striking out at my siblings while I was doing it. I learned early on that my brace was heavy and hurt when used as a club, and that crutches and canes caused great pain when I swung them and connected with flesh. I could punch and more. All my siblings still talk about the time my brother was messing about with me while I was at the kitchen table and I simply jabbed out with my fork and punctured a vein in his arm. The blood was everywhere, including in my eggs, and we kids were all stunned. My brothers and I were ten and eleven, my sisters in their early teens. Our parents didn't witness the incident and, as was often the case in our house, keeping this from them was paramount. We stopped the bleeding and applied a bandage, and he changed into a long-sleeved shirt. To this day, my brother complains that the tines of the fork were crooked and as a result his scar is too.

If dealing with my walking issues inside the home was complicated and at times difficult, outside it was even more so. I hated that children, both strangers and kids I knew and thought of as friends or potential friends, would imitate my limp, trying to provoke me into some reaction. When I did lash out in anger or attempted to catch them, they would run away laughing, safe in the deliciously guilty knowledge that I couldn't catch them no matter how hard I tried. I found schoolyards really tough and school kids at times really cruel, but for the most part I just sucked it up and tried to pretend it didn't bother me, though it did. I didn't want to be the whiny kid, the one who complained about every slight and insult.

I remember one gym class in grade five, after we had moved to Winnipeg from Calgary. We were playing soccer, a game I was ill-equipped to take part in. My classmates decided, unanimously, that I should be the goalpost. Goalposts don't move and limps aren't much of a problem if you're stationary. I took this badly, and when I got home I was distraught to the point of tears. My parents were distressed and did the thing parents often do: call the school and complain. It was a Jesuit school, staffed by priests and nuns, and they were tough. The next day, the teacher gave my classmates the parochial-school equivalent of hell. The students responded as any cowed group might, with overreaction, and voted me captain of the team, an honour I quickly declined given that it was even more ludicrous than being a goalpost. With the permission of my teachers, I proceeded to find something else to do with my gym time. Strangely, while the goalpost vote had made me feel sad and weak, the school solution left me embarrassed and ashamed. And I wasn't by any stretch finished with the nuns at that school.

Walking and limping had all kinds of effects on me growing up. Cub Scouts was a washout, but I always thought being an altar boy would be a slam dunk. In the early sixties, it was not unusual for a kid from an Irish Catholic home to entertain the idea of entering the priesthood. This career path set in early on, largely because having a limp didn't seem to be a barrier when it came to matters of faith. Becoming a priest, I thought, would solve a lot of problems: I'd win the admiration and respect of my parents, my grandparents and Catholics generally, and it was a job that didn't seem to have any physical fitness criteria. After all, does the Bible not say, "Behold, I am going to deal at that time with all your oppressors, I will save the lame and gather the outcast, and I will turn their shame into praise and renown in all the earth"? Some children spend their free time playing football; I spent a lot of mine pretending to be a priest. I knew that the first step in this process was to become an altar boy.

In Winnipeg, I started to put the whole project of my calling as an altar boy into action. I signed up at our parish church, which was run by Jesuits and located next to the school, so practice was easily attended on my way to or from school. I can still remember the excitement, the sheer joy of having this thing, this activity that could be mine but that was also indifferent to my limp and pleasing to my parents.

In the beginning, all of us, altar boys and families, were looking forward to the really big event: Christmas midnight Mass. It was going to be in Latin, with Gregorian chants, a half-dozen priests concelebrating and 150 altar boys assisting at the service. And the whole event would begin with a procession through the darkened church with the priests swinging censers, altar boys carrying candlesticks and the choir singing. I can still feel the chill of expectation five decades on. But it was not to be.

I came home one day from practice, where we had been rehearsing for the big event, and my parents told me they needed to talk with me. They explained that the Mother Superior had called and announced that I wasn't going to be allowed to take part in the procession or the midnight Mass because my limp threw off the symmetry. What if I dropped the candlestick, she'd asked, and no I hadn't done that but I could and so on. Mother Superior told my parents that she and the other nuns and priests organizing the event had concluded it would be best for me if my parents delivered the news. I can still taste the anger and humiliation, and it still brings tears to my eyes. I was devastated, but at the same time part of me was aware that my parents too were very upset, deeply torn between their sense of obligation as good Catholics and their anger as caring parents. I never went back to altar boy practice in Winnipeg, or anywhere else for that matter.

If the nuns taught me that my awkward gait was something I would never be capable of truly escaping or ignoring, my parents taught me that there were real limits to their patience and their understanding of what I was struggling with. Not long after we arrived in Winnipeg, I started to experience severe and increasingly frequent stomach cramps. The sudden onset of the attacks and the degree of pain were sufficient to cause me to bend over sharply and moan aloud. In addition, the stomach turmoil and nausea were such that I lost all appetite. My parents took me to the family doctor, who determined there was nothing wrong with me. He suggested that what I was experiencing was psychosomatic, that I was simply seeking the attention I had received during previous "medical incidents." He suggested I get therapy, see a counsellor.

My parents accepted the diagnosis but were reluctant to seriously take up the prescription of therapy; neither was a big believer in psychological theories. My parents, my father in particular and with true vehemence, would tell me that there was nothing wrong with me, that I was imagining the pain. I was told repeatedly that I needed to stop pretending and acting out. As you might expect, these conversations would take place most often at the onset or conclusion of yet another bout of stomach cramps. I was terrified by the anger my parents expressed every time I clutched at my stomach or rocked back and forth trying to ease the cramps. I was bewildered by their insistence that what I was convinced was real was just imaginary, an attempt to get attention, a selfish move on my part and something I had to stop indulging in. The attacks didn't happen only at home, but also at school. My parents talked with my teachers, who then understood that I was acting out, faking an illness, and treated my cramps and me accordingly.

After several more weeks of continuing bouts of stomach cramps and lack of appetite, and despite numerous lectures on my need to abandon this imaginary illness, my father took me to see one more doctor, a specialist in internal medicine. While we were waiting to see him, I had another attack. I remember the look of anger on my father's face as he insisted I give up this faking. He said that once we had seen this new doctor and the doctor had explained that there was nothing wrong with me, I had to shape up and stop this nonsense.

We walked into the doctor's office and sat down in front of his desk, and before he asked a single question about what was wrong or what the symptoms were, before he did a single test—he simply stared at me and then turned to my father and asked how long my skin had been yellow. My father asked what he meant and the doctor pointed out that I had a deeply yellow hue, that I was displaying yellow jaundice, most likely a result of having hepatitis. He did a few tests, took some blood and prescribed some drugs. He also explained that I was probably experiencing real bouts of abdominal cramping and pain and that my appetite was most likely deeply reduced. He ordered our family quarantined and tested, on the odd chance that I had an infectious form of hepatitis.

For the next couple of weeks, the entire family was forced to stay at home. I took medicine, my cramps abated, and my appetite returned. The quarantine angered my father, who was forced to be off work, and made the rest of the family mad as well. But I was truly relieved. I had started to believe the line that I was just inventing ailments to attract attention. I was really worried that I had become something of a child prodigy at hypochondria. I was also angry that what

I had been going through was only real if someone else said so. The other lesson I was starting to learn was that I needed to downplay everything related to my health. I began to believe that the best course of action when it came to pain and difficulty was simply to suck it up and move on.

9

THE EXPERIMENT
UNDONE

My family lived in Calgary for a couple of years, transferred to Winnipeg for less than a year, and then my father's company sent him, and by extension us, off yet again. In 1965 we were living in Fredericton, New Brunswick. My father was on the team that was building the Mactaquac Dam, a huge hydro-electric project about twenty-four kilometres upriver from Fredericton that would eventually supply about 20 percent of New Brunswick's electricity needs. Moving to Fredericton from Winnipeg had all kinds of pluses. For my parents it meant being on home turf, just a couple of hours from Dad's family, most of whom still lived in Grand Falls, and an hour from Mom's only sibling, a sister, who lived with her husband and family of five children in Saint John. That helped a great deal when it came to dealing with the reality of once again finding new schools, new churches and new shopping routines and moving into yet another new house for the third time in three years. It also meant having to find new doctors.

In addition to the general practitioner who dealt with the whole family's colds, flus and other routine medical matters, I needed to be connected with someone who was somewhat familiar with polio and who could deal with both the consequences and the required follow-up surgery flowing from the Calgary experiment. Finding me a doctor was always one of the first things that needed to be dealt with. In terms of timing and urgency, it should go without saying that the rest of the family had their own rightful priorities. When I talk about the ranking of my issues, it is purely personal, and though my siblings and I have never really talked about it, I have no doubt everyone else saw it differently.

Fredericton was a small town compared with Calgary, Winnipeg or the city and suburbs of Montreal, but it had what we needed to live a relatively normal life. We five children were scattered in a number of different schools, and for most of the year school and studies were what we did. We lived in a ranch-style bungalow on Montgomery Street with a fully finished basement. We had what I remember as a huge backyard. We all had friends from school we hung out with, we did the normal things kids did. But I still wore a brace most of the time, still walked with a noticeable limp and still felt largely an outsider, believing that everyone zeroed in on the limp as soon as they saw me and judged accordingly.

It had been three years since the surgery that was intended to accelerate the growth of my damaged leg, and while the changes were of course imperceptible on a day-to-day basis, the reality was that the discrepancy between the legs was disappearing and there was more of an evenness to my stance and less of a limp, though still the same hitch, to my walk. It was always the expectation that three years was the maximum the procedure could remain in place before the rewiring of my circulatory system would need to be undone and my leg returned to its prior state. The undoing was necessary simply because if the left leg was allowed to continue to grow at an accelerated rate, then it might actually outgrow the right leg, which would of course create a whole new set of difficulties.

The problem was that we had moved four thousand kilometres from where the experimental procedure had been done, and finding a doctor to do the new operation in Fredericton or elsewhere in New Brunswick or even in the Maritimes proved impossible. It was early days in the new Canadian health care system, and my parents and doctors engaged in numerous long conversations about where I might go to find a doctor and a hospital willing to perform the surgery and how this would be paid for. In the end, it came down to the only option available: the Montreal Children's Hospital, where a heart surgeon who dealt with children had agreed to take on the surgery.

My parents and I were anxious. Montreal was a long way away, but my father now had family and friends living there. My mother and I went to Montreal first, and my father would follow closer to the day of the surgery. The doctor and the hospital wanted me there a few days in advance for examinations and testing. As well, I was about to go on exhibit.

During the course of my life, I have presented some intriguing medical situations, and doctors and medical students love to learn from the unusual. I showed up in Montreal the recipient of an operation that only a dozen or so other people in the world had undergone, and now it was about to be reversed. While the cardiac surgeon reassured my parents that this was all going to be routine, my days in the hospital were filled with rounds of medical students coming by to ask a series of increasingly intrusive questions about pain, mobility, walking, the attitudes of others, my family's reactions to my surgeries, and a host of other issues that as a twelve-year-old totally perplexed and irritated me. In addition to the medical students, there was a seemingly never-ending series of visits by doctors who dropped by in ones and twos to examine me and pepper me with questions.

I was also X-rayed, measured, tested, probed and prodded extensively. At one point I was subjected to a procedure where dyes were introduced into the arteries and veins of my legs in order to record the normal blood flow of my "good" leg and the abnormal blood flow of my "bad" leg so that the surgical team would have a sense of how things were working before the planned operation and how things should probably look after the surgery. I remember it was very painful, the needles were large, the dye seemed to burn, and they had me biting into a piece of wood in order to quiet my near screams. It apparently never occurred to the doctors or students that I might be tense, anxious, uninterested in being a case study, unwilling to somehow be on display or cited as an example. There was no complaining to be done, or at least no complaint I could make that would be listened to. Oddly, that aspect of the practice of medicine hasn't changed much, especially in a hospital with a teaching function. One of the things you quickly learn as a patient in a teaching hospital is literally an object lesson.

Eventually the tests and the examinations came to an end and the day of surgery arrived. My parents arrived at the hospital that morning fully expecting the operation to take a few hours. In fact it took seven hours, and when they later recounted the experience to me, it was clear they were horribly distraught, scared and panicking. When the surgeon finally emerged, he explained to my parents that he had misjudged. The surgery had been seriously more complicated than he had anticipated. But, he reassured them quickly, everything had gone well, they had been able to rewire the circulatory system in my left leg, and blood flow in my left leg now matched blood flow in my right leg. Surgeons are endowed with incredible egos, for good and for ill. The one in Montreal who took on my case was both brave enough and cocky enough to believe that he could do it.

After the operation, there was a period of convalescence while stitches healed and my leg adjusted to increased blood flow. It meant that walking was again temporarily compromised and getting around involved wheelchairs and crutches and, of course, my brace. I still used the brace to compensate for weakened muscles and the problem of a drop foot, an inability to raise my foot due to muscle paralysis, which had never quite been dealt with, but there was reason to hope that I was now on the path to a relatively normal gait.

Back home in Fredericton, I had every expectation that my life was going to be pretty normal from then on. My legs were pretty much the same length, or at least within the statistical norm of variance that we like to think of as the average human body. One leg was still smaller, weaker and less flexible than the other, but it seemed at the time that all these issues were manageable. I was ready to be a normal kid, someone who had once had polio but had moved past that. Or if not past, at least to a position where polio was something that had happened to me just as it had happened to thousands of others, and, like them, I was coping as best I could.

For a brief period, life was all about school, holidays, playing with friends, bugging siblings. It was the mid-sixties and the Beatles were on TV, Bob Dylan was entering my consciousness, and I was having fun. I and other kids from the neighbourhood played pranks on people, discussed comic books, explored nearby woods and just hung out. I read a lot, indulged in seriously nerdy activities such as imagining reconstructing the Security Council at the UN and following closely the race for the moon. I still couldn't play baseball or ride a bike—the weakened left leg ensured

that those activities were never going to be things I did—
but that was okay, as I had other things that were my own
and I could feel that I was truly becoming myself. It
sounds clichéd, but at least as far as memory serves, life
was good.

PART

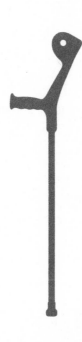

TWO

10

AN INNATE SKILL OR
A LEARNED BEHAVIOUR?

Learning to walk one time is pretty much enough for any of us. The reality is that those types of efforts, the learning of behaviours that will become automatic, require extreme dedication, energy, and brain and muscle power. I remember reading Marni Jackson's memoir *The Mother Zone*, and encountering for the first time the notion of maternal amnesia. It is the idea that after a baby is born, the mother loses all her memories of the trauma and the pain. She'd have to, or no mother in her right mind would become a mother for a second time. I remember thinking at the time and again years later that it seemed analogous to learning to walk. But of course, not all analogies are as simple or as apt as they might appear.

When my wife, Debi, and I were in Italy, we visited a gait research facility in Rome. While being shown around, I noticed what looked like the smallest treadmill in the world. It was no more than sixty centimetres in length, with hand-rails that were only about forty-five centimetres above the walking belt. It was a treadmill to test babies. They fastened infants as young as two months old into a safety harness and hoisted them above the treadmill, hooked them up to infrared sensors and recorded the child seeming to automatically mimic walking. I realized only then that mimicking walking was something I was very familiar with; I have done it to varying degrees all my life.

Simulators, where behaviour is mimicked, are at the leading edge of numerous learning environments, not the least of which is medicine. Imitating and practising behaviours can lead to concrete results.

People who study gait argue that much of what toddlers are doing is imitating behaviours they see all around them, carried out either by their parents and other adults, by siblings or even by other babies. The argument over whether walking is an innate skill is vigorous and ongoing, but the simplest answer seems to be both yes and no. Some animals, such as horses, are born able to stand and walk almost immediately. Humans are born without muscles developed to the point where the body can immediately hold itself upright, but babies do seem to have a "step reflex" from day one. Just as the work of Noam Chomsky in linguistics and language acquisition has provoked decades-long arguments about what is innate and what is learned, so too in the field of gait acquisition and gait development. What we can agree on is that perhaps there is something to the idea of Monkey See, Monkey Do.

Though we argue about the correct way to understand the origins of gait, how gaits develop, what constitutes an ideal gait and how gaits go wrong, there is some general consensus that gait is complicated and that most individuals are still maturing their individual gait even into their mid-teens. Through no fault of my own, I experienced a significant break in the process of gait maturation. I'm still dealing with the consequences of this unintended interruption in development.

We spend a lot of time, as a society, thinking about how we learn and the best way to acquire new skills. We spend significantly less time on how we lose skills and how we regain a skill once it is lost. In rehabilitation hospitals and clinics, especially with stroke victims, great progress is being made with new thinking about brain rewiring and skill reacquisition. When I was in my early teens, I learned some hard lessons about both those things.

11

THE UNOBSERVED HIP

The strangest things will cause me to flash back to when I was twelve. An acoustic ceiling tile in a doctor's or hospital waiting room, the feeling of plaster, finding myself in an awkward position with a leg bent oddly, being tangled in sheets, a closed bedroom door—all of these things often bring back deep, searing sensations of pain, confinement and loneliness, and sheer sweat-inducing feelings of panic, need and helplessness.

In 2007, I was appointed to the Board of Governors of St. Thomas University in Fredericton, New Brunswick. I had graduated from the university in the 1970s and it was an honour to be asked to serve on the governing body of my alma mater. On my first drive through Fredericton as a member of the board, my first time back in Fredericton in a quarter century, the car passed by 186 Montgomery Street, where our family had lived for several years. One look at that house and a flood of images poured in; frankly, many were deeply unpleasant and depressing. I asked the driver if we could stop. I got out of the car, stared back down the road and saw myself riding on a school bus and the bus hitting a pothole, which jarred me heavily. I remember getting off the bus and experiencing an incredible pain in my left leg. Leg pain wasn't unusual, but this was something very different. This wasn't an ache or a stab of pain—this was deep, nerve-crushing agony. Most of all, I remember the sheer panic and confusion for a brief moment at not being able to walk.

This moment came just a few months after I returned from Montreal and the major leg surgery to rewire my blood circulation. Standing on the road that day so many years later, I recalled the achingly deep anxiety I had experienced as I asked myself what could possibly be wrong now. I remembered being very, very scared. I remembered the looks on my mother's and father's faces when I told them what had happened, knowing somehow that this was what the question "What now?" looked like on an adult face. All of this and much more flooded back into my conscious mind that day in 2007 as I stood on Montgomery Street and stared up at the old house. I was remembering my lost year.

From my perspective as a patient, the most important thing that happens when I see a doctor is the diagnosis, the determination of whether there is something wrong with me that needs to be or can be fixed. I have been in a lot of doctors' offices, walk-in clinics and emergency rooms, and there are a myriad of ways that a diagnosis is reached. I have had a seemingly endless number of readings taken, and have been on the receiving end of all kinds of tentative conclusions. What I have learned is that diagnosis is as much an art as it is a science, and that means sometimes mistakes are made.

I have also learned through experience that when mistakes are made in diagnosis, there are a couple of key things that might have gone wrong: sometimes the doctor has leapt to the conclusion that something really rare is happening, and sometimes the doctor is experiencing tunnel vision and missing important signs. The tension of this dilemma, this problem of reaching or overreaching to an incorrect conclusion, was captured in the 1940s by a professor at the University of Maryland Medical School, Dr. Theodore Woodward, who coined the aphorism "When you hear hoofbeats, think of horses, not zebras." The implication, of course, is that the best bet might be to go for the more obvious conclusion, not the more unusual one. As with any aphorism, there is always an equally pithy and opposite saying to be found, and in this case it appears to be Hickam's dictum, coined in the 1950s by Dr. John Hickam of Duke University, which asserts, "Patients can have as many diseases as they damn well please." This is a very old argument, one stretching back to at least the late thirteenth century, when the Franciscan friar William of Ockham argued that when confronted with competing possibilities, choose the one that requires the fewest assumptions, a theory known today as Occam's razor. Just because a debate is an old one doesn't mean it doesn't continue to have real power or consequences.

I learned the harsh truth of both of these theories when I was thirteen and the doctors figured out why I was experiencing such extreme pain. I was stunned, my parents even more so, to learn that contracting polio had done more than cripple me; it had caused doctors, nurses and my parents to miss a very important feature of my birth. I had been born with a condition that could have been treated but wasn't, and now at thirteen I was about to pay the price of a missed diagnosis.

According to a number of sources, the idea of a congenital dislocated hip has been around since the time of the father of medicine, Hippocrates. Yet the disagreements about what it is, what causes it, how it is best diagnosed, how frequently it occurs and how best to treat the condition have given rise to hundreds of medical papers, dozens of books and some pretty extreme medical arguments. Despite the disputes, it can be said that around one in one thousand births involves "hip dysplasia or developmental dysplasia of the hip (DDH)," or congenital dislocated hip. It seems to occur most often with first births and with girls, frequently among Laplanders but rarely among the Chinese, or when one or both parents has experienced hip dysplasia. In essence, the dysplasia is a looseness of the hip bones, a tendency to dislocation or a form of abnormal bone growth.

I am not a Laplander, not a first child and not female, and neither of my parents had hip dysplasia, but I had been born with hip dysplasia. And yet no one noticed. The most generous explanation is that my doctors all made the same mistake. Once I was diagnosed with polio, everything about me was seen through the prism of polio. Pains, discomfort, tenderness, awkwardness and so on were clearly a consequence of polio; the impact of polio on my leg, the after-effects of treatment, the difficulty walking could be and were explained by the fact that I had had polio. It never occurred to anyone—or if it did, it was never raised—that I might have something else wrong with me besides polio; or, to paraphrase Dr. Hickam, I could and did have as many diseases as I damn well pleased.

Babies and infants have a more flexible and less solid body structure, and that can both create some diagnostic difficulties and improve the chances that once the diagnosis is made, remedial action is possible and quick. The medical literature is filled with guidelines about how the diagnosis should be carried out at different stages of the child's development and the corresponding treatment options available. Because there are often no symptoms, examination of the infant for hip dysplasia is normally done on a regular basis. The examination consists of bending the legs, flexing the legs, rotating the legs to see whether there are any indications that the ball and socket are not working as they should. If there are symptoms, they tend to include: legs that turn outward or appear to differ in length, limited range of motion, folds on legs and buttocks that are uneven when legs are extended and examined side by side, and delayed gross motor development (sitting, crawling and walking).

Such examinations tend to take place at birth, at six months, at under two years, and before six years of age. While not definitive, the literature suggests that if the diagnosis is not made before the age of six, just about every option except the most extreme measures is off the table. The bottom line for me was that it was not a case that hoofbeats were zebras, but that I had two different sets of hoofbeats happening at once. What was made very clear in the doctor's office at age thirteen was that "extreme measures" meant just that.

12

HIP SURGERY

A hip is a joint that looks a bit like a ball resting inside a socket. The ball sits atop the large bone in the upper thigh, the femur. The ball fits into a cup, or acetabulum, of the pelvis, and between them they create the hip joint. If there is a single focal point where all the mechanical elements of walking, standing, sitting and lying down come together, it is at the hip. So if there is a piece of your bone structure you don't want screwed up or messed with, it is the hip joint.

From the time I was born until I was twelve, I was moving through the world with a ball that didn't quite fit into the socket it was meant for, and the two were rubbing up against each other—grinding, actually—and wearing each other down. As a result, by the time I was twelve, there was no ball left and there was no socket left for the ball to fit into. For years, in addition to the sheer difficulty of walking with a shortened leg and paralyzed muscles, I had experienced a lot of pain in my leg—pain that I had been taught was just one of the consequences of having polio, having an unbalanced body and lugging around a heavy brace. Now I knew that some of the pain, some of the moments when walking was difficult if not nearly impossible, could be chalked up to the grinding of bone against bone that was taking place, minute by minute.

In 1965, hip replacement surgery in adults was still in the experimental stage. The first-ever recorded attempt at hip replacement is reported to have taken place in Germany in 1881. The more modern history of this surgery had its tentative beginnings in the 1940s in the United States, with an acceleration of experimentation in the mid- to late sixties. By the time the seventies rolled around, hip replacement had become common, if not as routine as today.

Today, hip replacements are common enough that they serve as a leading indicator of how well the medical system is treating older citizens. In 1965, however, faced with a twelve-year-old in need of a completely new hip, the orthopaedic surgeons of Fredericton didn't have a lot of options. They chose the one that seemed to promise the least onerous long-term consequences, though to be fair, the problem they needed to fix was the lack of a working hip, regardless of the long-term consequences.

A hip works when the femur is connected to the pelvis. If a ball-and-socket arrangement is not possible, then the second-best option, arguably, is to fuse the femur to the pelvis approximately where the ball and socket would have been. So that's what the doctors did for me. They moved the femur up against the surface of the pelvis and laid a silver plate across the femur, fastening it to the pelvis. I wasn't given any choice here. The surgeon sat behind his desk at the Victoria Public Hospital, with my leg X-rays up on a monitor, and laid out in clear detail what he and his team were going to do. There was no soft-pedalling the operation; he simply spoke in a calm voice about what seemed to him the only available course of action.

One of the things I knew then, and know with even greater certainty today, is that when you are beset with chronic conditions, life and medicine, health and healing take on different hues than if you are simply faced with a one-off condition or complaint. By the time I was twelve and facing hip surgery, doctors, surgeries and hospitals were so familiar as to be normal. I didn't treat these elements of my life as catastrophic; I just accepted that this was the norm, this was me, and this was life. It probably sounds cocky now, but at the time, checking into a hospital was something I just accepted as part of living. Of course I felt anxiety and shed tears, but I wouldn't express my feelings in front of others.

I went into hospital the day before the surgery and was prepped there for the operation. The night before surgery, I was alone in the dark, thinking about what was going to happen the next day. It was like the experiences I remembered having in Calgary and Montreal, stuck in a room by myself, trying to imagine how much tomorrow would hurt and what it really meant to "fix my hip." I was alone, and I was learning at twelve what it meant to be truly alone. In a room by myself, my parents gone home, my siblings at home, everybody going about their "normal lives," I was stuck once again in a hospital room. I spent hours on my back, staring at the ceiling, trying to figure out why I was so lonely and why this all felt so normal to me.

The evening before the surgery, I had an enema, and it was deeply, deeply embarrassing. I was in pain, afraid and uncertain about what was going to happen the next day. My food had been cut off, and during the last few hours before the surgery, the time in which I was supposed to sleep, I had to experience a deeply invasive procedure administered by a man I had never met before. Before bed, another stranger took my temperature and my blood pressure, gave me a sleeping pill and told me to get some sleep as they had a busy day the next day. The morning of the surgery, I was given another sedative and wheeled on a stretcher to the operating room. I was lying there, staring at the ceiling, feeling chilled and thinking, *How much is this going to hurt? Is this going to be like the other operations? Will my parents be there when I wake up? Will I wake up?* I went through the whole routine, which even at twelve seemed just that, a routine. I was lifted onto a table in a room with achingly bright lights and filled with people in gowns and masks. Needles were stuck in my arm, I was cold, a mask was put on my face, and a voice told me to breathe in, and then there was a taste in my mouth, a weird combination of medicinal and mechanical, and I was instructed to count down from 100 . . . 99 . . . 98 . . . 97 . . . and for the next several hours it was as if I were dead, no sensation, no pain, nothing.

While I was under, a long incision was made in my upper left thigh, in the area where my hip would once have been. After the leg and pelvis were exposed, the surgeon filed down some of the damaged bone, fixed the femur against the pelvis and fastened a silver plate to fuse the bones together.

The surgery is called arthrodesis, and in certain circumstances it is still used today, though much more often with ankles and wrists, largely because the rigidity that the procedure creates is more manageable when the range of movement being limited is relatively small—unlike the motion in a hip. A wrist fixed in position is by no means fun, but a hip and consequently a leg limited in their range of motion is a much more dramatic case. Today, the procedure would be used in a worst-case scenario where other possible strategies either had failed or, for some other reason, were not possible. In my case, it wasn't so much a worst-case or last-chance procedure as the only one available.

The other significant consequence of the surgery was that my left leg was shortened. After enduring the experimental surgery at nine years of age, and then the rewiring surgery at age twelve, the hip surgery wiped out any leg-lengthening progress and more. After the surgery, my left leg was nearly three inches shorter than my right leg. From the surgeon's perspective, there was no choice; no other options were available. From my parents' perspective, it was regrettable, a shame, but it was also what needed to be done. From my perspective, my once-normal legs were now a thing of the past.

13

A YEAR ON MY BACK

When I woke up from the surgery, in the recovery room, feeling the drowsy, nauseous, foggy mix of fatigue, weariness and just plain confusion often experienced when coming out from under a general anaesthetic, I really needed to pee. I was hooked up to monitors and an intravenous, but I threw back the blankets and tried to get off the bed to go to the bathroom. But I couldn't move. I couldn't lift my chest to sit up, I couldn't move my legs to the side of the bed. Why couldn't I move? Why was I like a block of wood?

A nurse noticed my agitation, rushed over and tried to calm me down. Even as a panicked twelve-year-old, I was able to prioritize. First things first: I told her I needed to pee. She got me a urinal, I peed. She rearranged my pillow, straightened my blankets, and took my temperature and pulse. I had two pressing questions for her: Why couldn't I move? And had the non-confidence motion in the House of Commons that day passed or failed? She laughed and, pulling aside my blankets, pointed to the plaster cast I was wearing that began just below my armpits and ran down my entire torso and my left leg to my toes. My arms and right leg were not encased in plaster. She said, "This is why you can't move."

I was stunned. The body cast was huge, heavy, and very, very white. I didn't know it at the time, but I was high on Demerol, a very powerful painkiller that had made me pretty much unaware of the cast while I was under the covers. In response to my second urgent question, she told me she had no idea what had happened that day in the House of Commons but maybe the doctor or my parents would when they came to see me.

That was me at twelve, encased in a body cast with a keen interest in politics. My problems with walking, my time in hospitals, and some natural abilities and inclinations had turned me into a reader. I loved the printed word and read anything and everything. I was also a news junkie, something that had begun when I was around six and has never abated. That body cast almost drove me crazy, and that love of reading kept me sane, as it always has.

There have been a number of points in my life when my experiences have changed me in so many ways, but none as much as the year after my hip surgery. I spent that year on my back, in that cast, confined to a bed in a room in our house on Montgomery Street in Fredericton. Getting into that room had required an ambulance ride up the hill from the hospital to our house and then being hauled on a stretcher through the front door and down a hallway to a room in the back. The attendants lifted me onto the hospital bed my parents had rented and I was home—sort of. It was home as I had never experienced it before.

I was often miserable, bored, anxious, frustrated and lonely, really lonely. My family didn't ignore me, but my siblings went out every day to school, to play, to hang out with friends. My father went to work every day and had chores on weekends and in the evenings. My mother, who was, oddly, my most constant companion, had a house to maintain and a husband and four other children to attend to. I was the guy in the back room and everyone would visit and talk, but none of it, none of that year, was the normal day-to-day life one experiences just being a kid in a large family going about his days, weeks and months.

I was constantly aware of being confined, both in a room and in a bed, but also inside the cast and unable to move. A task as simple as getting a book from across the room or picking a pen or piece of paper off the floor required asking for help. Everything deeply personal, such as washing, urinating, defecating, demanded that a family member, usually one of my parents, be part of the whole process. I was a twelve-year-old Catholic boy already angry with his body, and I had to share each and every bodily function with someone else. I was lonely and isolated except when I wanted privacy most.

I have never stopped wrestling with the chicken-and-egg question of how much of my personality and take on life have been formed by my experiences or, alternatively, to

what degree my personality helped me cope with my experiences. The year in a cast intensified that quandary, for from
that time right up to the present day I have always been prone
to the interior: I have an active imagination, and a high comfort level with being by myself and alone with my thoughts.
I am not saying I am my own best friend (there are parts of
me I dislike too much for that to be true), but I do, for the
most part, like myself and find that I can entertain myself.
During that year, I honed this skill. I told myself stories,
fully immersed myself in serial books such as Tom Swift and
the Hardy Boys, and allowed my imagination to range far
and wide. What choice did I have? If I hadn't let my mind run
loose and go roaming, I wouldn't have moved at all.

When I think back to that year, I realize that, to the extent
that a person's early adolescence is a critical formative period, much of who I am can be traced to a relatively extreme
confinement during which my major tools of survival were
books and my own interior self. If I had learned over the
years of family relocation that I had no sense of home and
that strange situations didn't particularly bother me, I
learned during the year of the body cast that I could be fairly
self-sufficient in terms of my mental survival. My confinement taught me what suffering, isolation and loneliness
can mean from minute to minute, day to day. Coming back
physically from a year on my back, learning to walk yet
again, taught me something quite different.

Ironically, in a story about learning to walk, lying still, in
a fixed position, plays a big role. I have since read that

dealing with being in a cast requires that the patient have lots of patience and a good sense of humour. Now you tell me.

I know at least two things about immobilizing part or all of the human body in a large cast (meaning at least the torso). First of all, the technique is not used often, and when it is, it is mostly with children, especially after "radical" surgery. It is deemed necessary in order to allow the body to fix itself, the thinking being that rest allows for connective tissues, muscles and bones to heal without inappropriate pressures or movements causing even more trauma. Secondly, immobilization can cause almost as many health problems as the injury requiring repair. It leads to muscle loss and degradation of tone, endurance, stamina and flexibility. Bedsores, infections and a lack of cleanliness are also seemingly inevitable. There is no way to disguise the fact that it is a messy, demanding and truly frustrating experience. And not just for the guy being immobilized.

During the year I was in the cast, I was in effect homeschooled, with much of the teaching, care, feeding and entertaining falling on my mother's shoulders. I know it was hard work for her, and it was a grinding experience for me. I was on the cusp of my teens, at times bored out of my skull, and emotionally ground down by what seemed to be a never-ending series of medical shifts and turns, experiments and unexpected developments. I was angry, demanding, frustrated. I was a handful.

In *Moonwalking with Einstein: The Art and Science of Remembering Everything*, Joshua Foer recounts some of what the research tells us about the way memories are formed and the way memories aren't formed. Part of the process is tied to the reality of new things happening; that is, something unusual takes place and the mind decides to remember it. In doing so, it creates a short-term memory that becomes stronger and more long-term the more often the mind reflects on it, or the more often we "remember" it. What aids in both the retention and the long-term strength of the memory are the various tags that become associated with it. Colours, smells, noises, emotions and so on all get tied up with a specific event or series of events. The trigger points for the recall or summoning of the memory become more varied and complex, and more likely to result in the memory being recalled.

So the key to memory formation is that something new has to happen. With certainty I can attest that when you take a twelve-year-old, put him into a body cast and place him in a bed for a year, time passes extremely slowly. In retrospect, the period is at best a blur and most often a blank. But I do remember some things with chilling certainty.

I know I could look out the window and see a tree. I looked at that tree a lot and watched it change through the seasons. That might partly explain why to this day I find trees so restful, and why I can spend hours zoning out by staring at a forest or even a group of trees. At the same time, I realize that there are all sorts of people who haven't spent a year confined to a bed who respond to trees in a similar fashion.

I know I listened to the radio, and it was listening to the

radio that started a lifelong fascination with and love of CBC Radio. There is something powerful about the medium of radio and the art of listening. For the makers of radio, the term "theatre of the imagination" is tossed around a great deal. I experienced this theatre first-hand.

If we're speaking chicken and egg, it was the tree, CBC Radio and reading that made me the person I am. Granted, the surgeries, the polio and the walking also shaped me. I listened to and paid attention to news, current affairs and information from a very early age. Sports never caught my attention, but stories of the United Nations Security Council and the goings-on over on Parliament Hill kept me rapt.

I also know that my routines were straightforward and dull. I had my own room, which was not normal in our house—the boys and girls were each in shared rooms—but in this case, given that I was in effect hospitalized, I was kept separate from everyone else. Imagine a house with two busy parents and four other children and a family room in the basement and the kitchen/dining room down the hall-way from the main-floor bedroom areas. In one of those bedrooms was me, and that's where I stayed for a year in a hospital-style bed with a trapeze bar that allowed me to pull myself up and shift around. I had a radio to listen to, library books to read and school assignments to do. I spent much of that year alone, ate by myself, largely entertained myself, and coped.

In time, the cast began to stink and I smelled regardless of how hard my parents and I tried to keep me clean. My mother sprayed can after can of Lysol. The stuff had been credited with stopping a cholera outbreak and was advertised as a preventive measure against all kinds of illnesses, a claim first made during the Spanish flu epidemic. I have no idea how many cans of the stuff I was responsible for my family going through, but I know that the smell still causes me to cringe.

It wasn't long after my year in bed that my mother began to grow seriously ill; in our family's communal memory, the two events are deeply connected. Massive doses of Lysol or bacterial contamination or simply the effort of caring for me while managing a household set off a chain reaction that created pain and suffering of a whole different order. Over the next fifteen years, she would deteriorate from a healthy woman in her mid-forties to someone in and out of hospital with mobility issues, severe and spreading arthritis, surgery for hip transplants, and a growing and evolving daily cocktail of drugs. As it turns out, my mother's physical deterioration would have eerie and difficult resonances in my own adult life.

My clearest memory of that entire year is the last day of my confinement in a cast. An ambulance came to our house and two EMS technicians put me on a stretcher and took me out of the room I had lived in for a year, down the hallway and through the front door, down a set of stone steps and into the back of an ambulance. For the first time in a year, I was seeing things other than the four walls of the room. We drove to the hospital and I was wheeled through the outpatients' clinic and into what is known as the cast room. My doctor and a technician came in and the technician used a power saw to cut through the plaster cast, stopping every once in a while to tear off chunks. In a relatively short time, the cast was gone. I just lay on the table feeling a very powerful absence. There was a coolness, lightness and ease all around me that to this day is a distinctly tangible sensation of freedom that I can summon at will.

14

LEARNING TO WALK
FOR THE SECOND TIME

When I sit for too long a period and then stand, there is a moment of deep hesitation. My left leg feels like a piece of wood, solid and immobile. I know the first step is going to be hard, and that causes me to feel a momentary, deep disappointment. That's not how I want it to be; I want to get up out of my chair and walk with total ease. After a second, sometimes longer, I laugh and realize that, regardless of how I want it to be, it is what it is. Sometimes, and it is impossible to predict why or when this happens, that sequence of disappointment and chagrin will summon up a very stark, harsh, pain-filled and somewhat embarrassing memory.

I am just past thirteen, only out of the cast for a few weeks, in a gymnasium that is part of the Victoria Public Hospital in Fredericton, New Brunswick. The gymnasium is located in the Fredericton Polio Clinic. The clinic opened in 1955 as a replacement for an earlier version that had over the years fallen into deep disrepair. Improving the facilities for treating polio patients had been a big election issue in

New Brunswick in 1952, and the promise by the Conservative Party to rebuild the institution may have helped them win the election. A community-wide fundraising effort and the overwhelming co-operation of the medical community turned the campaign pledge into reality in 1955. Then the success of the Salk vaccine in reducing the number of new patients meant that the clinic could turn more of its attention to rehabilitation. That's where I went after my year in the cast.

In this memory, I am standing between two parallel bars, with a hand on either bar. A woman standing outside the bars is telling me to take a step, and I cannot do it. She insists and I counter that it is too hard and I cannot do it. She tells me to take a step and I burst into tears, sobbing, my whole body shaking with a mixture of embarrassment, anger, frustration and a deep sense of hopelessness. I am learning to walk, I don't know how to do it, and all I really know is that I can't do it, though I also know that I have to. Not being able to walk is not an option; I have to get past this somehow.

That breakdown, those tears, that complete sense of inadequacy rest inside me today and simply form one part of my memory of learning to walk a second time.

Most people who have to learn to walk a second time have suffered some severe interference in their neuromuscular-skeletal system, and the relearning is more a question of rebuilding brain–body connections or damaged nerve pathways. Those were issues I would skirt later in life, but not when I was thirteen. No, at this point in my life my problems were of a different nature, but no less challenging.

The human body requires—demands—movement and exertion. Limbs, muscles, nerves, tendons and tissues not utilized properly will atrophy, and quickly. Recent studies suggest that muscle atrophy can take place at a rate of about 12 percent a week. After five weeks of non-use, 60 percent of the muscle mass and capacity can be gone. Tissue, tendons and bone also deteriorate the longer the system is immobile. Loss of bone density is particularly problematic. While new studies suggest that recovery can be quick after five to ten weeks of inactivity, longer periods create real remedial problems and long-term issues. So if a mere month or two of inactivity can seriously erode the body's ability to function normally, consider what a year means. Compounding all of this was the reality that I was still a youth, and youth is when the average person builds the muscle mass and bone density that will carry through into adulthood.

Put aside for a moment what relearning to walk entails and focus on the idea and the problem of rebuilding muscle, tissue, bone and tendons. Richard Asher, one of the great medical minds of the twentieth century, wrote, studied and practised in a variety of specialties. In 1942 he turned his pen to the question of confined bedrest:

> *Look at the patient lying alone in bed.*
> *What a pathetic picture he makes.*
> *The blood clotting in his veins.*

The lime draining from his bones.
The scybala stacking up in his colon.
The flesh rotting from his seat.
The urine leaking from his distended bladder
and the spirit evaporating from his soul.
Teach us to live that
we may dread unnecessary time in bed.
Get people up and we may save
patients from an early grave.

Overly dramatic, perhaps, but a graphic portrait of what I faced when I was released from my cast.

Once I was past the initial euphoria I felt when the cast was cut off me, the hard work began of trying to get my legs in shape and learn to walk again.

The problem my physiotherapist and I faced was one of sequencing. Rebuild the muscles and bone first, or start walking first? The reality is that it was not an either/or proposition; each needed to happen in tandem with the other. I needed to do exercises to rebuild my muscles so that I could start taking steps. Putting weight on my feet and legs would build up bone density. Building up bone density and muscle strength would make taking steps easier, which of course would keep the cycle going.

In addition to the loss of muscle, tendons and bone density, I also had the now relatively recent but at the same time old problem of one leg being significantly shorter than the other. What this meant was new built-up shoes, a new brace and a new internalized understanding of how my body stood and moved, as well as a new reconciliation of mind and body with the easiest point at which I could be both standing and at rest. This is a great deal harder than I make it sound. When I tried standing, I had to think about it a lot. It is difficult to explain to a person what they need to be doing when they stand. I have to find a balance point, a moment or a space when I am not swaying or in danger of tilting over. Once I find that place, I have to somehow figure out how to stand on just one foot while the other leg moves forward to a new place to stand, and then I am standing on that foot while moving the other leg forward. And now I am standing on both legs in one spot again and the whole cycle continues. This is a much more difficult problem than it seems. The key to all of this is balance and motion working together, and when one leg is shorter than the other, weaker than the other, it's a lot more complicated.

So there I was at thirteen, both trying to relearn what I had belatedly learned when I was a toddler and at the same time learning anew what balance now meant to me, what posture now meant to me and how I integrated these new understandings into a new series of lessons—all of this while building muscle, tendons, bone density and simple endurance.

Back at those parallel bars, I did eventually get to the space mentally and physically where I could walk, using the bars as a form of support. This meant that I could move my legs and traverse distance. It wasn't pretty, it wasn't easy, and it was very tiring, but having at least accomplished that, I could be fitted out with crutches and sent home. With periodic physiotherapy sessions at the polio clinic, I was expected eventually to reach the stage where I would be able to walk without the crutches.

15

USING CRUTCHES,
LOSING CRUTCHES

After conquering the basic steps with the physio-therapist at the polio clinic in Fredericton, I set about conquering moving around my house, going back to school and church, and connecting with what friends I still had after a year's absence. I had always found it awkward and slightly embarrassing to walk around with a brace and a limp. Re-entering the world with a new brace, a new limp and, on top of it all, crutches was just that much more emotionally painful. I lacked the voice to explain to my parents and siblings just how intimidating it was to be out among people, even the people in your own house, learning and practising walking, something everyone else so clearly did well and with ease. There was no outlet, no way to express the deep shame and awkwardness I constantly felt. In my family that just wasn't something you said aloud, or even whispered. My parents, my family, the Church and the world I grew up in all sent me the same message: suck it up and move on. Doing that meant getting rid of the crutches.

I used what are known as axillary crutches, the ones that rest just under the armpit and have a bar halfway down for the hands to grip. Today there are all kinds of crutches, made out of metals, woods and plastics, designed to address particular situations and the strengths and weaknesses of the person using the crutch. In the mid-sixties there were fewer options available.

The crutch is both a very old idea and a relatively new one. In essence, a crutch helps bear some of the body's weight and allows for the development of a gait that moves the injured or disabled individual from one place to another. It is not hard to summon up the image of a very early human using a stick or a branch in order to hobble along after a serious injury. We have all kinds of real and imagined images from wars and histories past of individuals using crutches to compensate for injured or deformed legs; after all, Tiny Tim hobbles around using a Dickensian version of the crutch.

The thing we immediately think of today when we hear the word *crutch* was first patented and commercially produced in 1915 by the French mechanical engineer Emile Schlick. But his design had several limitations, not the least being that it was a relatively awkward solid piece, rough and ready or expensively made-to-measure. It wasn't until 1945 that the axillary crutch, one that could be adjusted with screws and made to fit the height and needs of the patient, was invented by A.R. Lofstrand Jr., a Canadian. The amount of upper-body strength that the individual using crutches needs to use is determined by the design of the crutch.

With the axillary crutch, the focal point for the load bearing is the upper arms and chest; for crutches with cuffs around the upper arm or near the elbow, which I used on only a couple of occasions and never for long periods of time, the weight bearing is more distributed and less reliant on upper-torso strength.

My mother's father was a stevedore in Saint John, New Brunswick, who died before I was ten. I inherited from him the physiognomy of the barrel chest and very large and powerful hands. It does seem as if fate sometimes hands you what you need to cope with what it later throws at you. So even at thirteen, I could physically handle moving around with a set of axillary crutches.

At first, when I began using crutches, I moved with a lot of tentativeness. There was the whole problem of how much weight to put on my legs, both good and bad, and how much to bear through the crutches and my upper arms and chest. Added to the tentativeness was the very tricky issue of balance when I was still. Am I resting on my legs, am I distributing my weight through my chest, crutches and legs, am I feeling anxious and as a consequence tensing up? While walking, through all its phases, may seem simple and straightforward, requiring little thought, it is both slightly astounding and even more distressing to be made to realize how much thought, calculation, reflection, anticipation and awareness are involved in such a mundane and vital behaviour.

Just moving about the house was a good challenge for the crutches, and in addition we had school, church, and family visits with neighbours and relatives. It never occurred to any of us that activities would be structured around the guy with the crutches. I either took part or stayed on the sidelines, but not going was never an option; you weren't going to leave the guy with crutches at home alone.

One time that first summer after the cast had been removed, the whole family headed to southern New Brunswick, near Saint John, to visit with my mother's sister and family and some family friends who had a cottage by a lake. It meant a gang of kids, a gang of adults, some swimming, some fooling around with boats, sleeping in cottages, as well as barbecues and bonfires. I can still see the distance and rough terrain you had to cross to get from where the cars were parked to the cottages by the lakeshore. There were pathways and slight hills and stones and tree roots, all kinds of things to trip one up, and I felt an odd little stirring of pride that I was able to keep up and move where I had to move in order not to be a limitation or a drag on the rest of the family.

One night at the cottage, all the kids had been sent to bed and the adults stayed up to have a few drinks and talk by the bonfire. I found myself awake and listening to the conversation as the subject turned to me. I heard some of the adults express admiration and surprise that I seemed so mobile, and my father unexpectedly praised the two things I did well: move about on my crutches and answer correctly all the questions on the various TV quiz shows. I can still summon up the warm feeling engendered by his praise for my mobility and my brains.

I remember vividly the moment when I first walked without the crutches, months after the cast had been removed.
My brothers and I were in the basement watching TV. In
those days there weren't a lot of channels, and whatever was
on at that moment wasn't keeping us entertained. We were
fooling around, trading insults, dares, nasty comments and
probably a few shoves and fake punches. At one point one of
my brothers grabbed my crutches and took off running, and
I remember getting up off the couch and going after him,
moving relatively quickly under my own steam. My brothers
and I were just stunned: I could walk without crutches!

Yet another milestone passed, and this time unexpectedly.
In retrospect, I had probably been ready for some days, but
you do get dependent on established routines. And sometimes the only way to truly gauge the dependency and what
is necessary and what isn't is to take a gamble. In my case, I
was shocked, provoked and challenged out of my comfort
zone, but the end result was the same. I could walk without
crutches. I could walk.

My walking was stiff. My left leg was rigid. In addition to
little if any flexibility in the lower left leg, the movement of
my upper left leg was constrained by the lack of a hip joint.
Even when I wore a brace, there was a significant hitch on
my left side as I walked. When wearing running shoes, the
limp and hitch were even more pronounced. I simply figured that the limp was always going to be obvious, I was
always going to be stared at, I was always going to feel as
if I was the object of derision or pity, so I might as well

experience the sensation of freedom that the running shoes evoked. My gait eventually became an unconscious activity. In that sense I walked like everyone else, with little thought about what I was doing. Only occasionally, when stumbling or misjudging a distance for a short leg, or while experiencing joint, bone, muscle or tendon pain, was I once again reminded that I walked with a limp but, more important, *that I could walk*. In those moments I felt both sad and happy.

Not long after this, we moved for the final time as a family from Fredericton to Sydney, Nova Scotia, where my father had signed on to take part in the building of a modern coal mine. I was a teenager, and found myself several years ahead in school compared with others my own age. That was a consequence of having been put through an accelerated programme in Fredericton, during which I had done three years of schooling in two, and the Nova Scotia school authorities adjusting my grade level to account for provincial education differences. It was great in theory to put me into the grade that most challenged my abilities, but in practice it meant I was now an oddity in two ways: I had a serious limp and I was several years younger, and demonstrably smarter, than my classmates. It was nearly a perfect storm. I was awkward, embarrassed and uneasy throughout high school. I had no real friends. I had no real social life. I did have books, an insatiable curiosity and a deep drive to succeed at something, despite my leg.

16

SAINT JUDE

I love Aaron Neville's voice. I have listened to his albums for nearly thirty years, a provocative and moving mix of spiritual, soul and R&B. His rich, deep voice works well with joy, sorrow, hope and despair.

I suspect my mother and father never heard Aaron Neville sing, but I think if they had, they might have liked the sound. They were big fans of Harry Belafonte, Nat King Cole and Otis Redding and owned albums by all three, which I listened to repeatedly as I was growing up. We had this big stereo, one of the floor models that were popular in the sixties and seventies, with a turntable and AM/FM radio. I think they would have liked the way Aaron Neville could summon God, faith and hope into the hearts and minds of those who listened to him. They would have really liked his version of "Ave Maria," one of their all-time favourite hymns.

My mother would also have liked Aaron Neville's deep devotion to Saint Jude. The two of them would have had a grand old time discussing the patron saint of hopeless causes.

My mother and Aaron could have talked about the miracles that Saint Jude had made possible or the fact that Aaron wears a gold Saint Jude medal as a charm hanging from his left earlobe. The charm was a gift from his mother, who prayed to Saint Jude when Aaron was a young man caught up with drugs and dealing. My mother and Aaron's discussion would have been one that I would not have wanted to be present for; after all, I was one of the hopeless causes that Saint Jude supposedly had his eye on. I believe I was never supposed to know this, and when the truth was revealed, there was some embarrassment on both sides, but the chagrin didn't stop my mother from praying to Saint Jude on my behalf.

My mother had a Catholic prayer book that she always kept by her side, and as she aged, the frequency of her prayers increased. One of the most powerful and lasting images I have is of her sitting in her La-Z-Boy chair with the back reclining slightly and the footrest raised, hunched over the book, fervently semi-whispering the various prayers that she said every day, prayers such as this standard appeal to Saint Jude:

> O glorious apostle Saint Jude, faithful servant and
> friend of Jesus, the name of the traitor who delivered
> thy beloved Master into the hands of His enemies has
> caused thee to be forgotten by many, but the Church
> honours and invokes thee universally as the patron of
> hopeless cases—of things despaired of. Pray for me
> who am so miserable; make use, I implore thee, of that

particular privilege accorded thee of bringing visible and speedy help where help is almost despaired of. Come to my assistance in this great need, that I may receive the consolations and succour of heaven in all my necessities, tribulations and sufferings, particularly [mention your request], and that I may bless God with thee and all the elect throughout eternity. I promise thee, O blessed Saint Jude, to be ever mindful of this great favour, and I will never cease to honour thee as my special and powerful patron, and to do all in my power to encourage devotion to thee. Amen.

Sometimes, of course, if she was engaged in a novena, a nine-day cycle of prayers on the same particular cause, to the same particular saint or for the same particular person, she might mix up the prayers with something like this one:

O Holy Saint Jude! Apostle and Martyr, great in virtue and rich in miracles, near kinsman of Jesus Christ, faithful intercessor for all who invoke you, special patron in time of need; to you I have recourse from the depth of my heart, and humbly beg you, to whom God has given such great power, to come to my assistance; help me now in my urgent need and grant my earnest petition. I will never forget thy graces and favours you obtain for me and I will do my utmost to spread devotion to you. Amen. Saint Jude, pray for us and all who honour thee and invoke thy aid.

I remember when I first stumbled onto the fact that my mother was praying to Saint Jude for me. I was in my early twenties and visiting with my parents when I noticed the Saint Jude prayer cards lying next to her prayer book. I knew my "lives of the saints"; what good little Catholic boy doesn't? It just took me some time to piece together who or what the hopeless cause was. My mother was quite upfront about the fact that, short of a miracle, it was unlikely my legs would ever match or the pain would ever cease. So, as far as she could judge, there was only one other option. For her, my being freed of my physical burdens was the only way I would ever find happiness; my father was also convinced of this. That I disagreed or even that I thought of myself as relatively happy, doing work I enjoyed as a community organizer and engaging with friends I liked, was of no real account. Unfortunately for her own peace of mind, she was not around when I met and fell in love with Debi and became the insanely proud dad of Jane. Knowing my mother, she would simply have treated it as evidence of prayers being answered.

Saint Jude has always struck me as a weird saint, the embodiment of much that is wrong with prayers of desperation and the desire to see faith heal the ill, the halt and the lame. The reasoning seems to go like this: if you are sufficiently devout and worthy and can attract the attention of one of the saints or of Mary, the mother of God, and have sufficient faith, then perhaps—assuming God doesn't have some other purpose for your suffering—a miracle will occur and you will be cured. So when my mother spent hours praying for Saint Jude to intervene on my behalf, to make me whole, to make me happy, to take away my pain, she was creating her own trap of circular reasoning: either she wasn't or I wasn't or we both weren't sufficiently faithful, devout or sincere, or God had other reasons for my limping about in pain, or else I was truly hopeless, which meant of course that she should keep praying to the guy responsible for the hopeless.

Seeking miracles or magical cures, wishful thinking even, is not the exclusive domain of the religious believer; we can all fall into that trap. I clearly remember an exchange I had on this very issue while working on a documentary about post-polio syndrome in the 1990s. About half of all people who had polio experience a return of the disease, or more accurately a return of some of the most significant symptoms of the disease, decades later. I was spared that, but during the course of making the documentary I was asked whether I would take a pill if it could eliminate all the symptoms, all the consequences that had flowed from my contracting polio in the first place. I remember being stumped. After all, I am who I am because of what I have experienced. If significant parts of that could be eliminated, what would remain of my self?

To be truly fair to my mother and to put her prayers in context, the invocation of Saint Jude when a sick child is in need is a remarkably familiar reflex for Catholics. My mother meant well; she loved me, she prayed for me. It simply may never have occurred to her that it would bother me to be thought of as hopeless or so desperately unhappy that

I would require or desire an intervention of miraculous quality and character. And my difficulties with walking weren't always physical. As I learned from Saint Jude and then from the Buddha, sometimes my walking, or my problems with walking, had a flavour or quality that couldn't be dealt with in a physio session or with a cast, crutch or cane.

17

BREAKING MY FOOT
AND GETTING A BRACE

The human skeleton is perfectly capable of withstanding a lot of hard knocks. I know. Mine has been through a perfect storm, and for the most part it has rebounded as best it could, and really as well as could be expected. But at some deep level examined only late at night, I knew that age would inevitably wear and tear at what was already an imperfect and damaged structure. I feared, even if inarticulately, that the end result was going to be neither pretty nor easy. I had no sense of how quickly I would begin noticing the ravages of age.

The first harsh clues came when I was in my mid-twenties, living on my own in Sydney, Nova Scotia, and working as an outreach worker for a community economic development organization. Attribute it to my own life experiences or a BA with a double major in political science and philosophy, but I had latched on to the idea that helping create a fairer world was a way to help others and demonstrate my own intrinsic worth.

At that point, I had erected real psychological barriers

between my adult self and the kid with polio, the guy who'd spent a year on his back, the teen who'd found himself weeping at how hard it was to get out of a cast and back on his feet. I couldn't separate myself from that guy physically, but I could do it psychologically. All that was in the past, and if limping and shuffling was the price to be paid for getting on with things, limping and shuffling was what I would do. I had so many other things to attend to: school, work, reading, romance, and trying to understand a past, present and especially future that were connected to physical problems. Naturally, these thoughts were wrapped up, to a certain degree, with shoes.

At the time, I was relatively careless about the type of shoes I wore, as long as they were running shoes. I know now that by wearing sneakers I was putting way too much pressure and strain on a leg and a foot that were not in any sense capable of coping. But in my twenties and thirties, I rebelled against the confines of casts, braces, hospitals and doctors by simply ignoring just about everything that made medical sense. I wasn't death defying so much as damage denying. Spend hours, days, weeks, months and years weighted down, restricted in motion, wrestling with awkwardness, and you might get a sense of what I was pushing back against. At the time, though, none of this psychological behaviour was anywhere near the conscious level. I just loved the feel of canvas and rubber, and to hell with the consequences.

There were consequences. Breaking my foot was simply the most obvious one.

I remember the first time, walking with friends through Wentworth Park in Sydney and sliding down a small embankment and hitting the ground hard. I landed on my left foot first, yelping like a puppy, and then cursing as the shock of a sharp twinge turned into a bolt of the truly painful. Oddly, at this point in my life, one of the few things I had not done with my bones was break one.

Breaking a limb is not as easy as you might imagine, and that's a good thing. But it is easier to break a bone in the foot than in other parts of the body. There are twenty-six bones in the foot, and one in ten broken bones seen in emergency rooms is in a foot. There are five main types of breaks: complete, open, single, greenstick and comminuted. (There is actually a sixth, but it occurs only in children, something that never happened to me.) Depending on which bone is broken and how, symptoms such as swelling, pain and the ability to put pressure on the foot or even walk will differ.

That first time, I had what is known as a "single break" in the fifth metatarsal bone of my left foot—in essence, the bone that runs up the outside of the foot toward the little toe. I experienced all the normal symptoms: some swelling, slight discoloration, pretty intense pain, and limping—by which, of course, I mean limping more than usual.

Waiting rooms anywhere are slightly hellish, but waiting rooms in emergency wards are a separate type of hell all their own. Almost by definition, if you are in the waiting room of an emergency ward, you have a problem, and most of the people in the room with you will be in some form of agony and experiencing some degree of pain. At night, a number of individuals in emergency waiting rooms are intoxicated, which adds to the seeming chaos.

Until this point in my life, I hadn't spent much time in emergency wards, so it was a relatively novel experience. I am an intensely curious person, so I paid attention and learned about triage, shifting queues and the quality of patience that emergency room personnel need to both possess and display. And I learned something about equanimity and the lack thereof. Some people in emergency rooms think they are the highest priority regardless of the facts and insist on the same. Other people, me included, tend to accept that the professionals behind the glass have some sense of the relative emergency of each and every patient and are responding appropriately. Keeping that perspective is difficult, especially if you are in pain, but getting agitated or angry doesn't actually make things better.

After a few hours, I was examined by a resident, had my foot X-rayed and then took part in a conversation that has become a constant in my life whenever I encounter someone in the medical system. So, what's this scar? When did that happen? What was the nature of that operation? Where was it done? And so on, to the point where I can actually go on autopilot as I discuss all the ins and outs of my medical experiences.

On this occasion, the diagnosis was a broken foot and the treatment was a small cast, crutches and some rest. A few weeks in, the cast and crutches were replaced by a heavy-duty bandage, a cane and a return to running shoes. I believed that was that. I could not have been more wrong.

Over the next few years, I was to break my foot three more times, each time more painfully, each time requiring a cast or heavy bandages for a longer period. It was all of a piece with a growing and intensifying envelope of pain that was descending on my body. At first it was twinges and sharp pains in my legs, shoulders, hips, knees, ankles and eventually wrists. Everywhere I had a joint, I began to experience episodic and eventually regular and then near-constant pain. And sometimes this intensifying pain affected the way I walked.

I would get stiff, I would seize up to the point where it seemed as though my joints or limbs no longer worked, or at least no longer worked as I had come to rely on them to work. Sometimes, each and every step was extremely painful, and taking those steps became a matter of will as much as mechanics. Visits to doctors about the intensifying and widening range of pain produced a number of diagnoses, all centred on emerging forms of arthritis. One doctor observed that some forms of arthritis are induced through trauma and that the trauma my body had experienced so far had bordered on the extreme. As the pain worsened, my will actually strengthened. I was determined that my physical discomfort wasn't going to stop me, that I would continue walking and that I would simply push through pain as if it was simply a question of mind-brain-personality stuff, unrelated to physical phenomena or signals from my brain and body that things were possibly awry.

That stance was knocked for a loop when I was forty, after I had moved to Toronto. I remember the day very clearly. My daughter, Jane, and I were going to meet downtown and head to Queen Pasta in our neighbourhood to have a summer dinner with Debi. Jane and I connected on a subway line, and while we were waiting for a train, I was knocked over by a young woman pushing a baby carriage who was paying no attention to where she was going. I felt a sharp stab in my foot and Jane asked if I was okay. I said yeah and we headed off to meet Debi. During the meal, the pain in my foot just kept intensifying to the point where tears were pouring down my face. Debi drove me to the emergency room of the nearest hospital, St. Joseph's.

St. Joseph's is a hospital that attracts a very diverse clientele. Lots of immigrants with English as a second language frequent the hospital, a fair number of transient patients with no family doctor use emergency as a walk-in clinic, and as the evening unfolds the emergency room tends to fill with people who may have had a few too many drinks or sometimes are accompanied by police officers intent on keeping them in sight and in custody.

On an average day, the emergency ward at St. Joseph's receives 266 patients, the largest proportion of whom arrive at night. Any facility that busy naturally engages in triage; the most serious patients need to be treated first. That night there were a couple of guys who had been cut with knives in a bar fight; one slightly inebriated individual who kept insisting that his hand had been crushed when he slammed the storm door shut against it, something that appeared to confuse the attending physician and perplexed me as an eavesdropper; and a few folks who seemed ill with internal conditions and no obvious symptoms.

When my number came up, I was sent for X-rays of the foot and ended up with an orthopaedic surgeon who was doing an ER rotation. He studied the X-rays intently, did quite an extensive review of my medical history and had me walk a bit, as best I could. Then he started with the obvious: I had a broken foot. What mattered to him more was that I kept breaking the foot. He thought it was a problem of too much pressure on the foot from my walking style and my gait. Compounding the issue was a difficulty I was having with bone density and a calcium deficiency.

The solution was a brace. Twenty-five years after I had finally traded in the whole enterprise of binding up my leg and shoving everything into a built-up shoe, for the real and imagined freedom of sneakers, desert boots and relatively interesting footwear, this doctor whom I had never seen before wanted me to go back to a regimen that was buried deep at the heart of every nightmare I had. We all imagine what our future will be, and it is usually a mix of good and bad, hope and fear. My imaginings were deeply dark, focused on a decrepit and deteriorating bone structure with movement that was terribly limited if not impossible. I worried constantly that the helpless immobility that had been my year in a cast would be my inevitable future. When I heard him mention a brace, I was devastated, convinced that I was embarking on a repetition of my childhood: partial and then full confinement. In the seconds after he uttered that hateful word, I lived a series of horrific futures, each featuring an aged equivalent of a sad little boy rendered immobile by a cursed disease. Luckily for the doctor and for me, I may have nightmare scenarios popping into my head with way too great a frequency but I am also a fairly rational individual. I said, "Well, let's discuss it."

We talked at some length. His case was compelling. Because of the discrepancy in length between the two legs, every time I stepped down on my left leg, I was unintentionally doing so with greater force than I was using to move my longer right leg. And at the same time, I was never putting my full weight on my left leg when I was just standing, which was having an impact on both legs, and not to the good. He explained that the more damaged leg needed help just to do its job. So he wanted me to wear a brace with a ¾-inch built-up heel, in a shoe with a ¾-inch built-up heel. This would by no means make my legs the same length, but he figured it was a start and would possibly ensure that I didn't break my foot again. He put me in a walking cast while the foot mended.

The next few weeks were a hassle in terms of getting around; the full implications of living with what the doctor had ordered took a while to sink in. Once the walking cast was no longer necessary, I headed off to Toronto Orthopedic, where they measured my foot and leg in order to construct the brace. Constructing braces and made-to-measure splints has always been pretty much a small-scale manufacturing operation. Back when I was a kid, this type of work often took place in hospitals; in the nineties, the norm was that it was done in small clinics. Toronto Orthopedic has been around for decades, first in Buffalo and then, after the 1980s, in Toronto. Albert Pecorella founded the business in 1916; his great-grandson Daniel Pecorella runs the clinic today. For the Pecorellas, the business is almost artisanal and rooted in family.

When I arrived, I will admit I was not in a great mood and not looking forward to this procedure. I imagined that I would be repeating what I'd experienced in the 1950s and '60s. But the days of steel rods and awkward leather straps were over. In the 1990s they used a form of thermoplastic: they made a mould and then fashioned the brace out of superstring plastic designed to fit your leg perfectly. They built mine so that it extended from the tip of my toes and ran under my foot, encasing the bottom of the foot with a broad concave piece of plastic from my heel along the back of my calf to just below my knee. Instead of the heavy leather straps and buckles that kept my leg from sliding around in the metal braces, the Pecorellas used Velcro straps at the top and just above the ankle. On the plus side, the brace was significantly lighter than the ones I'd worn as a child or teen. On the minus side, the effect of a plastic form that hugged the shape of the leg was complete rigidity. I was undecided as to whether this was better or worse than what I remembered.

Getting the shoe was the other painful part of what I saw as a reversion to a previous state. Finding shoes that can be fitted with a built-up heel is not easy. A lot of shoes are made of a single piece, lacking a heel and sole that can be removed and reattached. Some companies have lines of shoes that can accommodate just that type of procedure. In Toronto there is a chain of stores that specialize in selling this very type of shoe and in retrofitting the shoes with built-in or built-up adjustments as per a doctor's orders. There's nothing wrong with these types of shoes, but they are never going to be featured in the style section of the newspaper. When people see you wearing them, they are going to leap to certain opinions about what kind of person you are. Shoes are shoes, and they all carried emotional baggage for me but it was baggage with little if any style.

So off I went to Foster's Shoes, a little store hidden away in a tiny outdoor mall surrounded by office towers adjacent to the subway entrance at Yonge and Lawrence. I dealt with a salesman who would continue to work there until 2010, and who had been selling shoes for Foster's almost as long as the chain had been in business. He was a meticulous and fastidious individual who could remember your name from one annual visit to another. He actually made the whole experience somewhat more tolerable with his attention to detail and his near-encyclopedic memory with regard to shoes, materials, potential problems and various brand benefits. He knew exactly what type of shoes I should be wearing, given the nature of the brace I would be using and the type of built-up heel, and I could think of no rational reason to object to his suggestions. So I walked out with orders for two pairs of basic black shoes, each pair to come with a built-up heel on the left. Though I was very pleased with the service and my new shoes weren't nearly as cumbersome as those I had worn in my youth, I will admit to feeling emotionally numb that day, as if in this seemingly lifelong war I was waging with walking, another battle had been lost. What I didn't understand then is that until the war is over, there is always another battle to be lost.

18

AN EARLY DEATH,
A HARD REMINDER

It's August 2012, and I am once again in a hospital waiting room. A slight woman who looks about my age sits alone in a corner and is clearly in intense pain. She slowly and continuously rubs her left hand down her left leg. In her other hand she holds a book she appears to be reading intently.

Faster than the wink of an eye, I am in a small room in a high-rise apartment building in Sydney, Nova Scotia. It is the late 1970s. Along one wall are two La-Z-Boy chairs separated by a couch. In a corner opposite one of the chairs sits a TV. In the chair farthest from the TV sits my mother, a slight woman, nearly sixty, clearly in intense pain, rubbing her left hand along her left leg and holding a book in her other hand. It's a Catholic prayer book and she is not so much reading as praying. Next to the chair is a small table and on the table is a TV remote control and a highball glass with a Tom Collins. It is early evening.

In the fifteen years or so that have passed since I spent a year lying on my back, she has gone from being a relatively hale woman to a state of frailty. She has extreme rheumatoid and osteoarthritis, her hips have failed and been replaced, her walking is difficult. She has had to use canes and walkers for some time and is for all intents and purposes housebound. As her children have gone off to lives of their own, her life has shrunk and become small.

I was not a good son. I visited, not as often as I should have, and my visits seemed to disappoint and irritate both of us. She worried about me and claimed I was impatient with her. She was right about my impatience. The drugs she took for pain and inflammation affected her hearing and her memory, she was constantly tired, especially at the end of the day, and she often fell asleep while I was there. But my irritation had nothing to do with any of that. Her downward slide was alarming to all her children, but especially to me. In addition to being alarmed, I felt a weird mix of guilt and shame largely because the start of her decline and my year in the cast were linked both in time and in causality. I was ill, she cared for me, she became ill, and so they were connected.

Watching her walking deteriorate so badly convinced me that I was seeing my future foretold. The pain, the immobility, the need for walkers and canes, the dependency on drugs to slow and make manageable, but not eliminate by any means, the degeneration and the pain—all of these combined to resemble and provoke my deepest anxiety. She was a model of determination, endurance and stout-heartedness in the face of all adversity and at the same time a harbinger of my future. And I could not escape the guilt that hovered like an aura around every encounter she and I had.

My mother saw the best of doctors and tried all the newest drugs and therapies. She had cortisone injections, gold injections and joint replacement operations, all of which provided some temporary relief but only delayed the inevitable. She took a medicine cabinet full of drugs, most of which required the taking of another pill to offset the side effects of the earlier one. The end results seemed to be simply foggy mental processes, tinnitus, stomach sensitivities, memory lapses and a certain ill-defined but real lethargy.

Without meaning to, my mother had become an object lesson. I might be following her path, but I vowed to resist taking the steps she took. I knew deep down that I would reject taking anything but over-the-counter painkillers, that anti-inflammatories were not an option until the side effects were more under control, and that if more surgeries were required for my leg, they would be put off for as long as possible.

When she died, at sixty, it was the consequence of an odd combination of medical confusion, diagnostic misstep and a body worn out well before its time. A nasty infection deep within an artificial hip was mistaken for a bad case of the flu and the medication used to reduce the fever masked the worsening infection. This was one more time in my life when hearing hoofbeats and thinking horses was clearly *not* the best strategy.

She was hospitalized, but within days the infection erupted and in essence fried her neural systems and left her brain dead. I was there with my father when he made the decision to remove her from life-support. As I watched my mother die, my deep-seated Catholic guilt made me believe it was only appropriate that I be there, given that I was the person putatively responsible for her physical decline.

I carried the vision of her too-early death and her extreme difficulties with walking through the '80s, '90s and 2000s as my own walking worsened and my own pain intensified. What we often forget is that our physical activities frequently have roots that are tangled up with our mental processes. Pain is physical, emotional and mental. Walking is learned behaviour mixed with habits both good and bad, built up over a lifetime. Tolerance levels, workarounds, "life hacks," in terms of our performance and endurance, are all behaviours that speak as much to who we are as to what we can do.

In the early 1990s, not quite a decade after her death, I experienced the first of what I came to think of as my physical breakdowns. That is an overly dramatic way of describing periods or bouts when simply walking was really, really hard, partly because of the pain but also because of stiffness and an odd sense that walking required more effort than I could muster on a day-to-day basis. When I got out of bed, it was as if my leg had become a block of wood or a piece of stone. I had to consciously think about how to take a step; it was as though I were thirteen again and standing between parallel bars. When I finally made the step, moved the leg from rest through swing to rest again, the pain involved was intense, shooting up the left side of my body, and then I would have to repeat the cycle.

I was living in Toronto's Annex neighbourhood when I experienced that first extended breakdown. It was a Saturday in December and the walking was wickedly difficult, the pain extreme. But I am a firm believer in Newtonian physics: a body at rest tends to stay at rest and a body in motion tends to stay in motion. I walked to a nearby underground mall both to shop and to force myself to move. Getting around the mall was excruciating and worse was running into people I worked with who were taken aback at how slow and stiff I was and how much pain I seemed to be in. They were quick to take their leave and I was left awash in embarrassment as well as extreme pain and relative immobility. It was another one of those moments when I was forcefully reminded of my mother and left near despondent about what my future might entail when it came to walking.

19

WALKING STICKS
AND SCARS

I n the umbrella stand by our front door, I keep an eclectic collection of walking sticks and canes. They are made of wood, carved and plain, of metal and of strong plastics, and I don't know exactly how a couple of them are constructed. Some fold up, some are adjustable, some are bespoke and some are one-size-fits-all. I bought one on Manitoulin Island, Ontario, one in Bellagio, Italy, a couple at a Shoppers Drug Mart, and several by mail order through a travel supply company. Each and every one represents a stage or phase in the chronicle of how my walking deteriorated in the 1990s and 2000s.

The one from Manitoulin is a modern version of an old-style Aboriginal walking stick I bought to help with uneven terrain. The one from Bellagio is a silver walking stick with an owl's-head top I bought to climb the convoluted and steep steps of the villages around Lake Como. The Shoppers Drug Mart canes came into my possession when I was experiencing my breakdowns and walking unaided was just too difficult.

For such hated things, the walking stick and the cane have a rather glorious and intriguingly metaphoric history. While the use or presence of the walking stick has often been a synonym for physical weakness and need, it has just as often been a symbol of power, authority, style and class. They have been made of every material imaginable and have spanned the range from dour and plain to remarkably ornate and even gaudy. Financiers, industrialists, generals, kings, prime ministers and gangsters have all used canes and walking sticks as emblems of control, strength, wealth and authority. Historians of the walking stick also note that the stick has been used as a weapon, an item of dress, a symbol of occupation and all of the above. There are apparently more than two thousand patents outstanding for gadget sticks that hide swords, booze, tobacco, money, drugs, telescopes and even radios. I have always secretly fantasized about a cane that doubled as a flask, but then I start wondering about booze and walking, especially when the walking is unsteady. There is a reason why a sobriety test involves trying to walk a straight line.

Adopting a cane made me confront some truly difficult issues. First was coming to grips with whether everything was figuratively downhill from this point on. Much of the disabled community likes to describe fully functional human beings as TABs, or temporarily able-bodied, stressing that all human beings wear down physically, some of us just do it faster than others. I remember at one point in the 1990s being asked by a boss if I objected to her putting me down in

a report as disabled given that the CBC was trying to assess
how diverse its workforce was. I told her I didn't really object,
but I was curious as to why the corporation wasn't counting
people who wore glasses or had pacemakers or artificial
hips. After all, those are simply three more examples of how
technology can be used to overcome a physical limitation,
just as a cane can be used to overcome a limp or a stiff, unco-
operative leg.

People have a lot of funny ideas about canes and walking
sticks, and when a person uses one for mobility rather
than status, there is shame attached. If you google "using a
cane," you get millions of hits and thousands of sites with
videos and written instructions on the ideal cane to use,
the best way to use it and so on. My favourite how-to site,
Ask Doctor K, who in real life is a doctor at the Harvard
Medical School, has a fascinating story that captures our
ambivalence and shame about any tech that helps us:

> I recall a patient of mine who, like you, had just under-
> gone a hip replacement and had been given a cane.
> When I asked him how it was going, he said it worked
> pretty well at home, but that he couldn't go out. I was
> puzzled about why using the cane should be harder
> outside the home than in the home. It turned out that he
> was simply embarrassed to be seen in public using a
> cane. "Canes are for old people," he said. So I taught
> him to use crutches. That way people might think he'd
> been skiing an expert trail in the Rockies! Since then,

> I've asked many of my patients facing hip or knee replacement surgery about their views on canes vs. crutches. A fair number (and not all of them men) much preferred the image of using crutches to using a cane.

When I first read that suggestion by the author of Ask Doctor K, I wondered whether it wouldn't be better to challenge the self-esteem problem itself rather than work around the question of cane or crutches—but then I remembered that self-esteem is a big issue for me as well. The mind and its sense of self is a funny rabbit's hole. I once explained to a large radio audience that in my mind I didn't limp, and that was the self-perception I carried around for so much of my life. In my mind, I was just a guy walking; I didn't feel as though I limped. That's why I hate the huge plate glass windows that are ubiquitous in large urban centres. My mind could fool itself all it wanted about whether I limped, but all I had to do was walk by a storefront and I instantly knew that I limped and realized that what I was seeing then was what other people saw all the time. Right after glancing into a plate glass window, I would be deeply ashamed and horribly shy. In some ways it was just the whole scar issue all over again.

I have a lot of scars, and I am shy about them. Scars are the equivalent of a library card index to the injuries done to and the mishaps experienced by the body. You can read much of a person's medical history through scars, and you can acquire a sense of medical progress by noting length, width, stitch style and healing rate of individual scars.

But of course scars carry much more than the weight of mere medical history; they are rife with emotional content as well. "He jests at scars that never felt a wound" is one of those great Shakespearean lines that I remember even when much of the rest of the Bard's oeuvre escapes me. It's from *Romeo and Juliet* and refers to the metaphysical scar left behind after a failed romance, but there is a deeper truth.

A dictionary definition hints at some of the complexities buried deep inside the word:

scar 1 (skär)

n.

1. A mark left on the skin after a surface injury or wound has healed.
2. A lingering sign of damage or injury, either mental or physical: nightmares, anxiety, and other enduring scars of wartime experiences.
3. *Botany* A mark indicating a former attachment, as of a leaf to a stem.
4. A mark, such as a dent, resulting from use or contact.

v. scarred, scar·ring, scars

v.tr.

1. To mark with a scar.
2. To leave lasting signs of damage on: a wretched childhood that scarred his psyche.

We have come to associate scars with bad things. Just like the shifting perspectives on canes and walking sticks, so too the story of scars shifts over time. Scars acquired in battle were sometimes badges of honour, denotations of experience and adventure. Scars can indicate intentional modification of the body, in ancient societies and primitive tribes especially, and now in some avant-garde parts of society where they are becoming a vibrant art form. One report on new trends in the art of scarring explained, "Scarification (intentionally scarring a person's body) started as a ritual act. In its first incarnation, as a tribal rite, it was characterised by big, broad strokes, thick lines, and chunky raised scars with a symbolic meaning but little fine detail."

For me, scars are what happens when one is forced to deal with things in and of the body going wrong, and they riddle my left leg. They are the history, to date, of my struggles with polio and hip dysplasia and their consequences, and each scar tells its own story, even if it is a story only I can read. Equally true is that scars are like a limp, visual indicators that you are or have been damaged. It does hurt to write that word—*damaged*—but I can't escape the reality that there is a booming business in the eradication, or at least the diminishment, of scars. There are dozens of over-the-counter medications, ointments and creams that promise to remove ugly and disfiguring scars. In addition to the patent medicine industries attempting to profit from the scarred, there are also doctors who use plastic surgery and laser technologies to

undo the natural process of scarring after an injury. In
2012, New York University announced that a group of its
scientists had "discovered a possible treatment aimed at
diminishing the overall size of a scar and improving the
quality of skin within a scar." One of the lead researchers
on the project, Bruce N. Cronestein, explained that "scars
can be disfiguring and, if extensive enough, can lead to
diminished function and quality of life."

Some scars are entirely emotional. In the winter of 2014,
the news was filled with stories of a study conducted by
researchers at the Boston Children's Hospital's division of
general pediatrics that demonstrated

> at any age, bullying was linked with worse mental and
> physical health, more depressive symptoms and a
> lower sense of self-worth. And students who reported
> chronic bullying also experienced more difficulties
> with physical activities like walking, running or
> playing sports. Our research shows that long-term
> bullying has a severe impact on [a] child's overall
> health, and that its negative effects can accumulate
> and get worse with time.

What struck me when I read about the study was that it
rang both true and false. It's hard to make general findings
applicable to individual cases. When I was in my early
twenties, I went to work in Ottawa in the head office of a
Crown corporation that engaged in advocacy and organizing

with the needy and disadvantaged. At the same time, a new hire from the west coast came on board. Nancy and I were about the same age and both of us had had our share of difficult encounters with the medical system. She'd had scoliosis, a severe curvature of the spine that demanded surgeries and physio almost as complicated as mine. I walked with a pronounced limp on my left side; she walked with a pronounced limp on her right side. We formed an odd bond based initially on this peculiar coincidence of pairing. We both broke into gales of laughter one day when walking out to lunch and realizing what an odd sight we must be, listing and limping in opposite directions. We had both experienced bullying as children, and I suspect we both suffered from some diminished sense of self-worth, but we could commiserate as equals, so the self-worth issue was cancelled out between us.

Years later, Nancy and her spouse purchased a farm in the country and were raising sheep. I went to visit, and one day as Nancy and I were walking in a field, we encountered a neighbour of hers. She had told me about this fellow, a man who didn't believe a woman, let alone a "cripple," could farm. Then the neighbour's brother was made a paraplegic in an accident and had required all kinds of specially designed equipment to continue farming. Nancy believed that this need to accommodate a "cripple" in his own family was changing the man's perspective on things.

Nancy and I stopped to chat with him and the conversation turned to how bad farming was that summer, how the weather was terrible and the demands on farmers to compensate physically for the conditions were much worse than normal. He could not help but notice that I limped as badly as or worse than Nancy, and he became very self-conscious about his vocabulary, struggling to find words that might take into account our disabilities and those of his brother. We could have taken pity and moved on to other topics, but we didn't. He would pause in mid-sentence and you could tell by his eyes that he was looking for a neutral word to describe someone who had mobility issues. At one point, Nancy looked at him and said, "Gimp," and his eyes widened and he started to sweat and shook his head, and then I said, "Cripple," and his face turned beet red. We finally told him we were just kidding, that neither word was acceptable, and for a moment I believe he realized what it might actually be like to be on the receiving end of bullying. And I experienced again what it was like to bully.

I have to accept that my physical scars are what they are. It would be a lie to suggest that I don't care what others think because I do, but I believe my vanity and sense of self-esteem are rooted in issues deeper than mere scar tissue. My walking problems are tied up as much in the emotional as the physical, perhaps more. Mind you, it is easier to be relatively blasé about physical scars when they are on your leg and you don't wear shorts.

20

PAIN AND BUDDHISM

I have always had a hard time with an idea captured in this one quote from the American Buddhist nun and teacher Pema Chödrön: "Pain is not a punishment, pleasure is not a reward."

I am in a relatively dark hall, sitting on a straight-backed chair, my feet on the floor, my hands nested one inside the other on my lap, and I am watching my breathing. "This is me breathing in . . . this is me breathing out . . ." is how the repetition goes. Every few minutes I hear a voice calmly suggest that the mind will wander off and all that is necessary is to note that the mind has wandered to planning, to worrying, to judgment, to dreaming or simply to being lost in itself. Having noted that, simply return to following your breath. So it goes.

And then my leg begins to ache, throb, burn and blister. And each time the pain flares up, my mind and memory go down the most intricate and atrocious pathways, replaying embarrassing moments and a litany of occasions when I have felt betrayed by my body or betrayed others because of the torment my body was putting me through. I see myself snapping at strangers, yelling at friends simply because the pain in my leg, hips, shoulders, knees or wherever has robbed me of the very patience and tolerance we need to use with others. I remember not being able to enjoy concerts, movies, visits to art galleries or simply a meal with a friend or neighbour because my body's pain levels denied me any iota of pleasure, or simple conviviality.

I try simply noting the pain and going back to my breath; I try attending to my pain, attempting to understand its flavour and intensity, and then returning to my breath; but none of it seems to be working. I am still at the stage where I am looking for the workaround that will allow me to meditate despite the pain. But there is no workaround, and as I sit I feel as though the left side of my body has become a raging fire. I feel immersed in a horrid pit of memories all tied to being truly and deeply inadequate. Tears begin to flow.

I am in a small meditation hall, taking part in a Buddhist retreat in the Hockley Valley, north of Toronto, and at the moment I am simply trying to stay sane despite the pain. After what seems like an interminable amount of time but is probably five minutes, a gong sounds and our teacher tells us it is time to breathe deep, relax. The next meditation session is not for an hour and practitioners are free to walk about the grounds, practise yoga, engage in walking meditations, have twig tea or simply be. The key, of course, is to do so in silence. All the other meditators stand, bow slightly and leave the hall. I slide off my chair and lie on the floor, almost in a fetal position, as the pain in my leg escalates.

I lie there, not quite sobbing. The pain I am feeling is deeply charged and seemingly more than the pain I cope with every day. After about a half-hour, the extreme elements of the pain abate and I stand, take a deep breath and head outside. I think to myself, well, just forty-eight more hours and I am out of here, and then, if that pain happens again, I can at least moan aloud. Silent retreats demand a certain John Wayne–like true grit.

I first started meditating in Halifax, where I knew a fair number of the Buddhists hanging around the *Shambhala Sun*. When I moved to Toronto, Debi and I eventually became more intense practitioners, though searching for the right means, group and schedule for meditation has always proven to be a challenge. One of the reasons I stick to it is simply that it allows me to keep a clear perspective on my walking, my pain and how those two things affect my sense of self. The dirty little secret of every encounter with a health problem or the medical system is that no one likes to talk about the social and psychological aspects of being ill, experiencing pain, limping or simply struggling to walk. One thing Buddhists know and attempt to deal with is how much the characterization of the self gets caught up in and twisted throughout with each and every aspect of our day-to-day lives. We can use any aspect of life to somehow convince ourselves how special we are. My pain, my limp, come to define me, and I can use them to beat up on myself, to distinguish myself from you and others, or even as the reason why I can't be happy. This is not an insight unique to me.

On this particular weekend, one of the instructors is Tara Brach. She's a big-shot American Buddhist out of the Washington, D.C. area with a couple of bestselling books and a very good track record as a teacher. I have decided that this weekend is the time when I will finally talk with someone who might help me deal with the fact that I find life difficult because I limp, I am in pain, and these two things have worn me down for far too long.

One of the reasons I am attracted to Buddhism is for its at times distinctly non-Catholic approach to the reality of pain. Rather than wrestling with notions that pain might be offered up as a sacrifice to God or that God never gives you a burden too heavy to deal with, Buddhist teachings and Buddhist practitioners have a much simpler, more fundamental understanding. As the Buddha once wrote:

> *When touched with a feeling of pain,*
> *the ordinary uninstructed person*
> *sorrows, grieves,*
> *and laments, beats his breast,*
> *becomes distraught.*
> *So he feels two pains,*
> *physical and mental.*
>
> *Just as if they were to shoot a man with an arrow and,*
> *right afterward,*
> *were to shoot him with another one,*
> *so that he would feel*
> *the pains of two arrows.*

Or, in a less poetic sense, mindfulness guru Jon Kabat-Zinn writes: "Physical pain is the response of the body and the nervous system to a huge range of stimuli that are perceived as noxious, damaging, or dangerous. There are really three dimensions to pain: the physical, or sensory component; the emotional, or affective component—how we feel about the sensation; and the cognitive component—the meaning we attribute to our pain."

The Buddha says that most people shot with an arrow experience damage and injury from two arrows. The first arrow is the physical arrow that pierced the skin, drew blood and damaged the body. When that arrow is removed, the damaged tissue is cleansed, stitched up, bandaged and given rest time for healing, and within a reasonable amount of time the healing is done and the wounded individual is better. But the second arrow still hurts; it is the one that assigns blame and defines worthiness. It's the arrow that suggests, "If only I had been a better soldier, this wouldn't have happened"; "If only I were smarter, more attentive, braver, more agile, then I wouldn't have been wounded and caused stress and problems for my comrades"; "If only I were a better person, if only . . . if only . . ." The damage done by the second arrow is very difficult to heal. My polio, my leg, my walking, my pain are all deeply tied up in the two arrows: the physical damage done by disease and treatment and the emotional echo that continues to reverberate.

In some senses, my turning to Buddhism to somehow find a way out of the hold that walking and pain had on my life was not that different from my mother's search for answers and solace in Catholicism. The reality is that pain is a big stumbling block for all religions. Every morning, I tackle a Buddhist insight such as this one from Ram Dass: "There is grace in suffering. Suffering is part of the training program for wisdom." There is wisdom there, insight, acceptance and resignation, as well as a possible way out. But it is also remarkably similar to the idea of offering up one's pain to God as a sacrifice. Depending on the moment, it sounds smart and makes sense or appears to be an exercise in pure masochism. Much of my adult spiritual life has been about trying to parse that difference between smart and sensible and pure masochism.

The meditation weekend where I spent far too much time lying on a floor and moaning in extreme pain was horrible, yet it illuminated a new way of approaching the world.

The routine of a silent Vipassana retreat is relatively straightforward and consistent. I got up early, meditated, walked to the dining hall, ate, and then engaged in a bit of manual labour and helped clean the kitchen. After the work detail, I meditated, listened to a dharma talk, meditated again, walked to the dining hall and ate, meditated, took part in small-group sessions with our teachers, meditated again, walked to the dining hall and ate again, attended an evening meditation and talk, drank some truly horrible twig tea, and then tried to sleep. Sleeping was hard. I was sharing a room with two other guys and they snored (I suspect I did as well), and it is hard to communicate the displeasure that snoring provokes without breaking the silence. Bright and early the next day, a gong sounded at five-thirty, and I and the forty-five other people who had committed the time and money to take part in the retreat ran through the whole routine again. Every retreat, including this one, has a theme, and the thread running through these four days was the Buddhist idea of loving-kindness, for yourself and for others.

During one of the small-group sessions where participants could break the silence to raise issues that might be hindering efforts at meditation, I raised the issue of my pain. Beverly, one of the Buddhist teachers that weekend, suggested that mindfulness was all about paying attention to the things, big and small, in our life that were claiming our attention at the moment. She explained that believing you could meditate only when conditions were perfect was simply one more trick of the self to put off the task of deep and true attention. I nodded but still wondered how that applied to my attempts to meditate in a dark hall while half my body seemed aflame and all my mind was deeply distracted. She went on to say that rather than try to find ways of putting the pain aside, I could just allow it to wash over me without judgment and without effort, to accept myself in that moment. Again I nodded, and again I wasn't sure how this might work.

But I did try for the next two days simply to note the pain. Whenever memories and emotions emerged to attach themselves firmly to the pain, I would, as per the advice, simply note that I was judging or projecting or planning or regretting and return to my breath. By no means was this a lock on the problem, but at least it helped me avoid the fetal-position agony I had experienced on the first day.

Vipassana meditation retreats often emphasize walking meditation. In fact, meditators switch from sitting to walking and back again throughout the course of however many days, weeks or months the retreat lasts. At one level, this is perfectly reasonable. Days upon days of simply sitting can cause physical difficulties; walking allows the body to stretch and move. Of course, for me, my rather imperfect walking was also painful and led me to ruminate as opposed to meditating on the past. On the other hand, and in ways I did not ever anticipate, walking meditation also made me think about and contemplate how one does walk. To be mindful, the purpose of the retreat, I had to attend to what I was doing at the moment, because that's what mindfulness is. Breathing, washing the dishes, cleaning my house/room and of course walking were all opportunities to ground myself in what my life is about. Walking meditation demands that I watch, that I see the raising of my leg, that I am aware of swinging my leg forward, conscious of lowering my leg, and I pay attention, real attention, to following through with my foot as my other leg rises and the pattern continues. For a time at least, my mind is deeply in the present and I get at least a momentary insight into the constituent elements of my walking, and how imperfect and painful those elements are.

The advice Beverly had offered about simply observing the pain where it arises, its nature, its intensities, its shifting from place to place was equally applicable to walking. As I have mentioned, over the course of my life I have become a connoisseur of pain, and this exercise of observing the pain, without judgment or emotional footnoting (both very, very difficult tasks), proved to be fascinating. The pain while sitting and the pain of walking were truly different. It was definitely more difficult to sit. But walking brought many more memories and recriminations to the fore than sitting did. There is a phrase I internalized as I grew up: "you can't win for losing." It seemed that weekend to be most truly apt. The retreat centre was in the heart of a valley and had deep strands of woods and long walking paths through high grasses and thistles. As I walked through these quiet natural patches, I realized that I wasn't experiencing the romantic notion of hiking through the woods or strolling through meadows or fields. I find walking on uneven ground awkward. I am clumsy at it. I stumble, trip, lose my footing and sometimes fall. All of these work together to remind me that I feel inept at the physical, that I am most comfortable with the cerebral. Within minutes I am spiralling down memory holes where relationships have failed because I am too logical, not demonstrative, too word fixated, too little touch oriented. Watching my legs rise up, swing through and come down may be a great way to centre myself in the moment, but it is also a seductive way to lose myself in nasty self-flagellating memories. It also gave me a number of opportunities to note that I was judging and many many moments to return to my breath.

Eventually the retreat came to an end. Coming out of silence was strange. I was most perplexed at how quiet we all were, as if everyone in the room was as reluctant as I was to actually talk. Being quiet is unusual for me, and yet I didn't want to be free of the rules that had kept me silent. I felt sad that I was re-entering the world where noise, buzz and external distraction were the norm. Over the next few minutes more and more people began to speak and the teachers encouraged us to ask questions both in the large-group setting and individually. I took advantage of that and approached Tara Brach to ask about the thing most on my mind: how do I get past, or lose my attachment to, my pain, my limp and my medical history? The conversation went like this:

PK

I need help learning how to meditate while in extreme pain.

TB

Everyone who meditates needs help doing it while under stress, worried about work, worried about their kids.

PK

Yeah, but this pain is real, it physically hurts, it isn't just a stress thing.

TB

How does it hurt? Can you describe it?
Describe just the pain, not the thoughts or
emotions that go with it, just the pain.

PK

Well, I guess it depends. The pain in the
ankle is different from that in the knee or
the hip area. Sometimes it's just a lot of heat,
sometimes it feels like grinding—but it really
distracts me! It flares up and I start thinking
about being a kid or that time when—

TB

Just the pain? Is there a colour associated
with the pain? Is the pain in your ankle or
knee or hip constant?

PK

A colour? Wow, I am not sure about that, I
could try and note that. But it isn't constant,
the pain is always there, or seems to always
be there . . . but . . . not in one spot all the
time. But it just distracts me terribly, it
sends my mind down pathways and I have to
keep pulling it back.

TB

When you are meditating, do you get distracted by hunger or thirst? Are you sometimes sleepy and go into a dreamlike state?

PK

Of course, but none of that is like the pain. . . .

TB

Why is hunger different than pain? Aren't they both physical distractions, in the sense you mean it?

PK

Sure, they are both physical, but the sensation of being hungry will fade away, the pain doesn't.

TB

Are you sure? You said the pain shifts, sometimes it is in the ankle and sometimes the hip, and you said the pain wasn't the same in both, so does one type of pain fade away and another comes into sight?

PK

You mean like hunger or tiredness or other emotions?

Back and forth we went, parsing out exactly what I thought I was experiencing when I said I was experiencing pain and why I thought pain was so distracting. We engaged with how pain works or seems to work, the linkages between pain and experience, pain and memory, pain and judgment. Most importantly, we discussed how pain wasn't me and I wasn't pain.

Tara Brach is no stranger to suffering, pain, loss or emotional turmoil. Among the many reasons she is a bestselling author and much in demand as a teacher is her keen and clear willingness to use her own struggles to illustrate the challenges and opportunities, the drawbacks and real benefits, that the mindful life creates.

What she told me that day was both simple and extremely complex. There is a cartoon summary of the bottom line of most religions, and the bottom line of Buddhism is "Shit Happens" (which is distinctly different from Catholicism's "If Shit Happens, You Deserve It"), and what we all forget is that "shit happens" to everyone. The key to applying this to one's own life is to understand that pain occurs, suffering is inescapable, and what really grinds us down is the belief or hope that if only our particular pain were gone from our lives, then life would be grand. So as long as I believe that a limp, a shortened leg or extreme pain is the only thing that makes my life less than it should be or could be, then to that extent I am letting my pain, my leg and my limp define me and my life.

Mark Epstein is a Harvard Medical School–trained psychiatrist and the author of a couple of fascinating books on Buddhism, medicine, pain and suffering. In an essay entitled "Shattering the Ridgepole," he laid out what for me is the real difficulty in what I was trying to accomplish:

> As the Buddhist view has consistently demonstrated, it is the perspective of the sufferer that determines whether a given experience perpetuates suffering or is a vehicle for awakening. To work something through means to change one's view; if we try instead to change the emotion, we may achieve some short-term success, but we remain bound by forces of attachment and an aversion to the very feelings from which we are struggling to be free.

21

YET ONE MORE
HOSPITAL VISIT

I have a love-hate relationship with the art and science of medicine.

On the one hand, I have been saved more times than I can count. I have liked most of the doctors and nurses I have dealt with over the years. But on the other hand, I have spent way too much time in waiting rooms, clinics and doctors' offices, having X-rays, ultrasounds, imaging, blood tests, and stool, mucus and urine samples taken, measured and recorded, to be anything but jumpy when once again I have to see my doctor.

By my late fifties, I had achieved some sense of equilibrium in my life. I had a good job as a producer with CBC Radio. I wrote, taught and lectured in my spare time. I was part of a loving family with a gorgeous house in the west end of Toronto. I was in pain and walking was not easy, but there seemed to be something of a balance between the things that wore me down and the things that made me smile.

But in June 2011, I was feeling remarkably rundown. I had no energy. My walking had grown stilted and almost shuffling. At times I found it really hard to breathe and other times I could hear the blood pouring through my body and it frightened me. I went to my doctor and said I was feeling out of sorts. He told me I didn't look good. He wondered aloud about my pancreas. He ordered blood tests and sent me for some imaging of my stomach and intestines at a clinic across the street. He admitted he had no idea what was going on. I was very scared.

The next morning, June 21, at around seven o'clock, the phone rang. It was my doctor and he told me to go to St. Michael's Hospital right away and tell the admitting personnel at emergency that "my doctor told me to come and that I had a hemoglobin of 47." I had no idea what he was talking about, but there was no mistaking the urgency in his voice. On the way to the hospital, I used my iPad to figure out what hemoglobin levels are and what the problem might be. In essence, hemoglobin level is a measure of the number of red blood cells you have. Red blood cells carry oxygen throughout the body, and the fewer you have, the less oxygen is distributed. The less oxygen, the bigger the problem.

At the hospital, I did exactly what my doctor had told me to do and within about thirty seconds a doctor came around the corner, looked at me, motioned me forward and told me to lie down on a bed. He had a nurse take blood and said he would be back shortly. About ten minutes went by and the doctor and nurse were back. He told me he'd had to check the hemoglobin level for himself and he had confirmed that it was indeed at 47. He explained that he had actually never seen anyone with a hemoglobin that low who wasn't a corpse, let alone someone who had come into emergency under his own power. He said he'd be back, and then the nurse set up an intravenous and started a blood drip into my arm, opened up a clipboard and started asking about my medical history.

"It's complicated," I said.

In my twenties, in addition to breaking the bones in my feet, I ended up spending weeks in a hospital in Ottawa suffering from a severe, almost fatal depletion of the chemicals in my body. All the calcium and sodium had somehow been leeched out of me and my bone marrow had stopped producing white blood cells. I was convinced then that I was going to die and my doctors shared my fears. I was extremely lethargic and for the longest time was convinced that my body had betrayed me yet again, this time for good. The doctors who treated me, including the chief hematologist on call the day I went to the emergency room, took risks and pushed limits to restart my bone marrow system, and the gamble worked. It was months before my body was anywhere near back to normal, to the point where I could return to work.

In my forties, I was misdiagnosed with colon cancer and spent a really dreadful few weeks convinced I was going to die. It turned out that what the doctors thought was colon cancer was actually a diseased appendix, but we only discovered this after surgery to remove the colon cancer, a very serious form of surgery. The panic I had been feeling about dying was misplaced.

Now here I was, in June 2012, once again seemingly
confounding the entire medical staff of a hospital. Oddly,
that can be and often is a good thing, what my family and
I call the "House Effect," after the television show *House*, in
which the main character, Dr. Gregory House, solves medical conundrums that befuddle every other doctor on staff
in the hospital. Doctors are like those in any profession:
much of what they do each and every day borders on the routine. So when a person walks in with a problem or symptoms
that challenge them, throw them for a loop or simply seem
impossible, they become engaged.

What I knew was that I was exhausted. What the doctors
knew was that my symptoms were such that I shouldn't be
alive. Their first tentative conclusions weren't reassuring.
Once I had been admitted, a team of three doctors gathered in
my room. The lead doctor on my case told Debi, Jane and me
that he thought I had a particularly aggressive blood cancer,
adult leukemia, and he wasn't optimistic about my chances.
I was stunned, Jane burst into tears, and Debi lost all colour
in her face. The doctor did note that he was an oncologist and
that his mind tended to work that way, and said that another
member of the team, a hematologist, didn't agree and she had
a number of tests she wanted to run. So he was willing to sus-
pend his judgment for twenty-four hours while tests were
done. In the meantime, they were going to continue to give
me blood in order to try to boost my hemoglobin.

Luckily, coming to a conclusion in line with the thinking of the hematologist didn't take as long as the story arc

on *House*. The tests revealed that, for whatever reason, my body would not absorb vitamin B12. There is a protein that combines with vitamin B12 so that it is absorbable into the bloodstream, and my body was treating it as a foreign body to be destroyed. Vitamin B12 deficiency can lead to megaloblastic anemia, which had brought me to the edge of death.

Vitamin B12 is one of the most important vitamins the body takes in, and a lack of B12 can affect the nervous system, short- and long-term memory, energy levels, breathing and a number of other vital functions. As the doctor and I talked about the problem, I remembered that pernicious anemia was something my mother had suffered from and that she used to keep little vials of B12 in the fridge and would have shots on a regular basis.

The simple remedy for me was monthly injections of B12. The doctor kept me in the hospital for a couple of days, did a few more tests (he was a thorough guy) and kept the blood transfusions flowing as well as ordering B12 injections to boost my levels.

The last evening before I went home, he dropped by my room and we talked. He and I had hit it off and he was curious about my medical past. We talked about B12 deficiencies and he told me the fascinating history of the problem. First identified in 1849, pernicious anemia perplexed the medical community and was a fatal disease. Two of the big focuses of research were how the human body could actually turn on itself in such a deadly fashion and what remedial options could be tried. The best minds in the area of blood research were engaged with the problem, with few concrete results until the 1950s, when injecting B12 directly into the bloodstream was tried. With such a simple solution available, research into the problem itself stopped. Now, there is a resurging interest in the problems associated with B12 deficiency because of our aging population. Over time the body can lose, partially or fully, its ability to absorb vitamin B12, and some researchers are beginning to suspect that the increasing incidence of dementia among the elderly may actually be the result of a vitamin deficiency.

My hemoglobin emergency ended happily but also reinforced my slightly divided sense of appreciation/dread regarding all things medical. I remember that first night in the hospital before the medical team had reached any firm conclusion about what was wrong with me. I was in a semi-private room. The other patient, an elderly man in the grips of a severe case of Alzheimer's, spent the night caught in a seemingly horrible series of memories, and every fifteen minutes or so he would engage in a period of howling and moaning, repeating a phrase about how cold he was and muttering a name and asking where she was. I was hooked up to a blood bag on an intravenous, anxious—scared out of my wits, actually—about what the morning would bring, and my roommate's delirium was just making everything that much harder. I was awash in memories of hospital stays as a boy, as a teen, as an adult. Hospitals make me feel lonely, helpless, abandoned by those who love me—silly overreactions that, while not grounded in reality, had me on the edge of tears. Lying on the bed, hooked to a bag of blood, unable to sleep, conscious of every passing minute, I realized this was the future I most feared. In the light of day, the worries retreated to the edges of my consciousness—not vanquished or banished, just set aside for the moment.

Little did I realize that the four days I spent in hospital being diagnosed and set on the road to recovery, and the few weeks I spent rehabilitating and boosting my hemoglobin, were just a dress rehearsal for a much more complicated medical adventure.

My parents, Cyril and Thelma, on their wedding day.

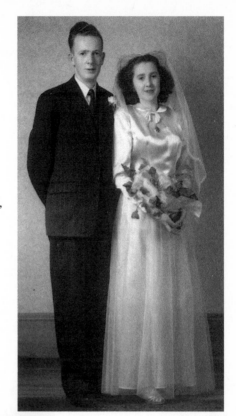

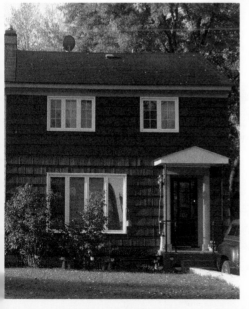

Our former house in Deep River, Ontario. The photo was taken recently; the house looks much as it did in the 1950s.

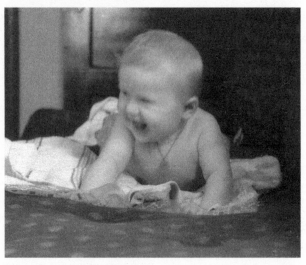

Me at five months, for all appearances a healthy baby.

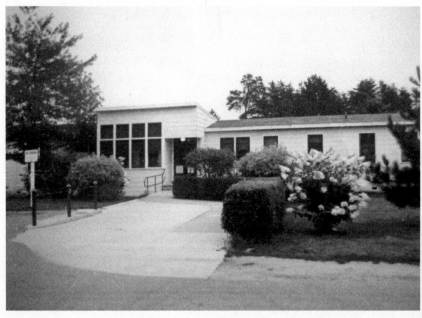

The hospital in Deep River, Ontario, the first of many hospitals in my life.

All of the family together in Deep River in the early 1950s. From left to right: Mary; me; my father, Cyril, holding John; my mother, Thelma, holding Paul; Kathy.

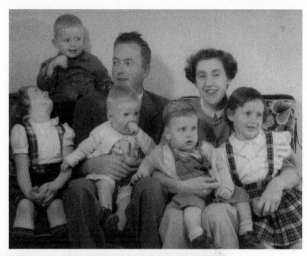

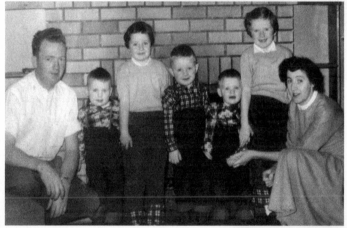

Our family in 1959, in our home in Buckingham, Quebec, one of the many homes I grew up in.

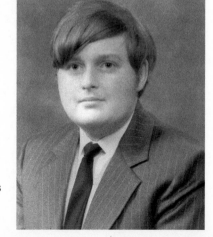

Me in 1966, in my last year of high school in Sydney, Nova Scotia. I was as nerdish as this photo suggests.

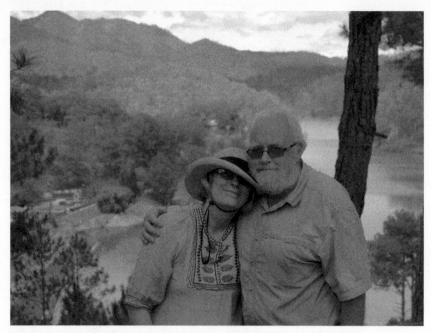

With my wife, Debi, in Vietnam, at the Valley of Love, on our last trip before the surgery in 2012.

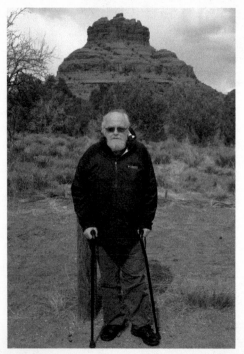

Our first big trip, eight months after my surgery in 2012, and I try hiking in the desert near Sedona, Arizona.

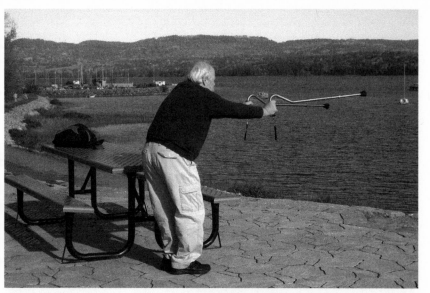

Back in Deep River in 2013 to see where it all began. I take the opportunity to exercise.

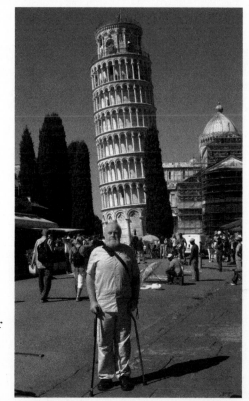

In front of the Leaning Tower of Pisa in 2013. One of us has been made straight.

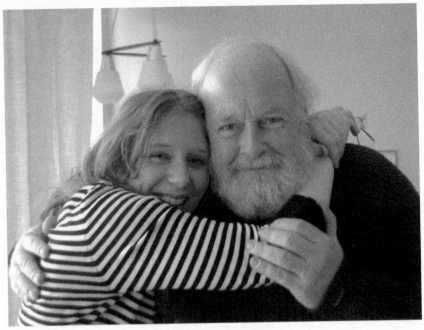

My daughter, Jane, always a shoulder to lean on.

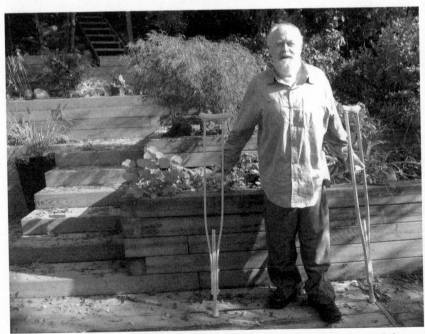

After the surgery, standing straight and tall for the first time in my life.

PART

THREE

22

ME AND MY HIP,
YET AGAIN

In January 2012, Debi and I travelled to Vietnam. Walking was at times difficult there, but more because of terrain and really lousy sidewalks than anything else, though I did experience a more than usual amount of stiffness and soreness on a daily basis. Vietnam is a gorgeous country that still bears significant wounds and scars from its nearly thirty-year war of national liberation, not to mention another twenty years of economic isolation. The Vietnamese people were warm, friendly and, with a few notable exceptions, pretty much indifferent to our presence as tourists. They had their own lives to live and were neither aloof nor obsequious with the Westerners who moved about in tour groups or on their own, as we mostly did. The exceptions were in true tourist locales, where the odd beggar was more the norm than elsewhere.

The other exception, and at first it was truly odd and irritating, was the number of times Vietnamese people would stare at my limp and shortened leg. It isn't as if Vietnamese society is devoid of people with physical disabilities; in fact, just the opposite. It is a country still reeling from the ravages of the application of Agent Orange as a defoliant by the US military, a weapon of war that damaged the genetic structure of generations and has resulted in many deeply deformed individuals. Some of these victims are actually "on display" at the entrance to the War Remnants Museum in Ho Chi Minh City.

So why the intense, invasive stares? Perhaps they assumed I was old enough to have fought in the last phases of the Vietnam War and wondered if I was one more of the "War Tour" Americans reliving their youth; perhaps I had been injured in the war and that was the cause of the limp. Or maybe it was just curiosity about why I hadn't taken advantage of the power of Western medical technology and had my leg fixed years ago. Every time I had a conversation with a Vietnamese person, the belief that people from North America had access to the best food, medicine and opportunities was clear. The stares didn't affect me the way stares did when I was a child. I didn't feel that humiliation, it was more a mix of shyness and confusion, as if they were suggesting my limping somehow didn't compute. Though I wasn't embarrassed, I was constantly reminded that I did limp, that my walking was awkward.

A couple of days after we returned to Toronto, I experienced a sharp, overwhelming spasm of a new type of pain, severe enough to make me gasp. Intermittent flashes had become the norm, a polish, so to speak, on the backdrop of near-constant agony that was my daily experience. But this was something different, something that worried me. The next morning I got out of bed to go to the bathroom and as I took a step, a similar spasm shot up the inside of my leg straight into my pelvis. For a moment I could not move. I hopped a little and then everything was normal again; I was back to my default reality, the usual low-grinding pain.

Back home from Vietnam meant returning to work at the CBC. I loved my job, and getting to work was for the most part not difficult: a five-minute walk to the subway station, a twenty-five-minute subway ride, first on an east-west line and then the north-south route. Finally, there was the five-minute walk from the subway to the CBC building. Normally it was a breeze. But now, not so much. My left leg ached with every step. The crowded subway seemed to drill into my skeletal structure. And on too many days I was exhausted by the time I made it to the office. Over the next few weeks the situation worsened. The sharp spasms right up the leg into my pelvis became more frequent. Even worse, as far as I was concerned, was how frequently I heard myself gasp out loud. Showing signs of distress embarrasses me—I like to see myself as tough, impervious. Hearing myself gasp or suck in breath at the intensity of the pain was a whole new experience. It frightened me. Was my lifelong dread of hard, inevitable degeneration coming true?

My GP often makes me laugh. One time I complained about feeling a persistent numbness in my right arm upon waking and he asked me if I slept on my side. When I said yes, he told me to calm down about the numbness or learn to sleep on my back. He went on to say he had the same problem and if he could cope, so could I. My visits to his office always include some talk about politics and the world as well as the state of my health. He has guided me through a number of very strange medical problems over the past fifteen years and I literally trust him with my life. When I explained that the pain levels I was experiencing were extreme, even for me, and that I needed some sense of where I was at and what I could expect, he didn't waste time. He sent me for imaging of my leg and hip.

Sitting in the large waiting room at the private imaging clinic across the street from my doctor's office, I felt both relieved that I was taking steps to figure out what these different symptoms might mean and also anxious about the forthcoming explanation for the intensifying pain.

About a week later, my doctor and I met to talk. He explained that from what he could tell, the silver plate fixing my femur to my pelvis was carving striations into my pelvis and that the femur appeared to be dislocating, or sliding in and out of position. He looked up at me, half smiled and said that in his professional opinion both those factors might well be the reason I was experiencing the extreme pain. It was delivered deadpan and with a touch of arch humility. If what he was saying was true, of course that's why I was experiencing this intensifying agony. He's a general practitioner, and a specialist might need to be brought in to make it official, but sometimes a thing is so obvious that once it is spelled out you can't help but agree. He explained that the next step was to see an orthopaedic surgeon and, while he was just a GP, it would be his bet that my future involved yet more surgery.

I have a dark side and often smile at difficult juxta-positions, anything with a tinge of existentialist dread mixed in with sheer ultimate futility. I hate surgery. I hate pain and the deterioration in my walking. But if surgery is the remedy for the aches and the problematic walking, then surgery it is. The diagnosis assured me that there was a strategy available, a course of action. That is the thing about extreme pain: it is a touch more bearable when there might be light at the end of the tunnel.

Getting to see a surgeon took a tough and taxing three months. I used a cane all the time and the agony that was moving grew worse. Sleep, never my strong suit, became even less steady, deep or restful. Debi tells me that for most of the time she has known me I have moaned and groaned in my sleep and that during this period it became constant.

Getting to and from work was harder with each passing day. My pain and the sheer weariness from walking were turning me into a short-tempered grouch. I snapped at colleagues, friends, even Debi and Jane. I kept hoping that acerbity was rooted in the pain and not in some deepening tendency toward curmudgeonliness. I was anxious that I had stopped being a nice guy. For everyone on the receiving end of my impatience, moodiness and simmering anger, it didn't really matter whether all that nastiness was physical in origin or the result of a souring personality. But it mattered to me. All of this agony was stealing my sleep and robbing me of the things that made the pain tolerable: work, reading and companionship.

23

A DIAGNOSIS,
A PRESCRIPTION

Toronto Western Hospital is a huge facility covering an entire city block on the edge of the inner core of the city. It got its start in the late 1890s when a group of doctors banded together to create a hospital on the western rim of the growing city. Today it is part of the University Health Network, a group of four teaching hospitals associated with the University of Toronto Medical School. Thousands of people stream in and out of it every day, and though the hospital is known for neurosurgery, it also does much in the areas of orthopaedics, arthritis, rheumatism and other related bone, muscle and tendon illnesses and diseases. This is where I go in June 2012 to meet with Dr. Khalid A. Syed.

I am told in advance to bring water and something to read while I wait in the orthopaedic clinic because the window of my appointment is three hours. With iPad in hand, water in my bag and Debi to talk with, we wait almost the full three hours before we are called into an examining room. There we meet a young woman, a medical student doing a surgical rotation and assigned to Dr. Khalid Syed's team. She and I do the now-familiar "brief" medical history. I give her the CD copy of my X-rays and she inserts it into the computer and pulls up the images of my hip. She has me lie down on the exam table and move my legs: spread them apart, lift, flex, move the knees, bend the foot, roll the hip, indicate the pain centres, and on and on.

After about fifteen minutes of this, she leaves to fetch Dr. Syed. The surgeon walks into the exam room followed by three people, the medical student we have just spent time with and two others. Syed is a remarkably polite individual, an old-school gentleman. He smiles, says hello, asks how both Debi and I are. He apologizes for the long wait and exudes the sense that he is there for the two of us and that he has all day. He introduces his team, then listens carefully as the medical student tells him about all the tests she put me through and points out the images of my hip that she has brought up on the computer screen. Then he pretty much asks me everything again while looking at the images and lightly moving my leg. He asks about the pain a lot—where it is and how it has changed over the years. We talk a bit about his background, his studies at the University of Toronto and his fifteen years of surgical work at Toronto Western. I have of course googled him and I ask about some of his research, especially his studies into the effect of music on post-operative recovery.

After about ten minutes of this back and forth, he explains that the first difficulty is that I don't really have a hip, and he will have to build one. Then he has to try to remove the plate that fixes the femur to the pelvis and create a ball to sit atop the femur. He muses about whether there can be any lengthening of the leg to diminish the discrepancy slightly, while he is building the artificial ball for the new hip, but then says it's a tricky issue because I might suffer nerve damage if he gets it wrong. He talks about titanium versus ceramics and explains a bit about how my age figures into the calculations. He asks where I got my X-rays done, and after I tell him it was at a private imaging clinic, he says that if we proceed I will need to have a new set done at Toronto Western because he needs full access to the X-rays, which he wouldn't have in the case of X-rays done in a private clinic. Basically, he is running the possible scenarios by me and asking if there are any questions. I have a few, but I have done my research and have a pretty good idea of what is what in this conversation.

There is a lot of language around legs—*stand straight, stand tall, get a leg up*—as well as a lot of social and sexual status around height and bodily symmetry. We talk about attractive people being a tall drink of water, but we never think of a lack of symmetry as a plus. Culturally, the image of the lame and halt, the gimp and cripple is used either to depict individuals worthy of pity or to describe situations of intense difficulty or severe shortcoming. Hearing something described as "lame" or "crippling" almost always sets my mind racing, and I experience a weird mix of shame, anger and humiliation. The rational part of me has never learned the trick of keeping the emotional part in check.

Dr. Syed's musings about the possibility of lengthening my weak leg brought back painful memories of the failed attempt when I was nine to make my legs the same length. Needless to say, the experiment I took part in as a child didn't work out well for me. The idea of trying to accelerate the growth of a shortened leg was just part of a spectrum of ideas that were being experimented with in the 1950s and are still being experimented with today. Leg lengthening is a form of surgery that is complicated, controversial and deeply enmeshed in the history of orthopaedics.

According to the most recent statistics, nine thousand people from around the world go through a leg-lengthening procedure every year at the Ilizarov Centre in Kurgan, Russia, named after the surgeon who invented the most common lengthening technique. Another five hundred undergo similar surgeries in the United States. One doctor who has performed many of the operations described the process as follows: "You gradually stretch out the healing bone sort of like salt water taffy." Of course, getting the bone to grow is one thing. Once the legs are the same length, the patient needs to relearn how to do all those things one does with a leg: bend the knee, turn the ankle, flex the foot and walk. I can attest that none of that is as easily done as it is said or written. And if it doesn't go well, "unlucky patients can suffer complications such as multiple fractures, scarring, an off-kilter gait and arthritis as well as hip, knee and disc pain."

But none of this is what Dr. Syed was musing about. He was so cautious about the possibility that I didn't really give it a lot of thought.

The big issue on Dr. Syed's mind is when to do the surgery. He asks if I would be willing to wait five years. He is trying to figure out the optimum point in my life to do hip surgery. The younger I am when I get an artificial hip, the greater the chance I will need a replacement one before I die.

I tell him that in Cape Breton there is an expression about "going spare," meaning going crazy. I then say that if I had to wait five years and the pain and deterioration of walking continued or worsened, then I would go spare. He smiles and says he understands. He asks me what I expect from the surgery. I tell him if I can do what I did earlier in the year— travel to Vietnam and walk about without difficulty—then I'll be good. Again he smiles and says he gets it. He tells me his assistant will give me a date for the operation.

Dr. Syed's assistant books me in for August 24, a little less than two months away, schedules me into a day-long pre-op session at the hospital in a month, gives me a very thick binder of instructions and sends Debi and me on our way.

24

PRE-OP

Two months seems long yet is no time at all.

I was working at a job I loved, it was June and we had a great deck on which to while away the summer nights, Debi and I had plans to go to plays at the Stratford and Shaw theatre festivals, and Jane was getting ready to return to school in September. Life was busy and pleasant. But under all that, I was still experiencing harsh pain, I wasn't really sleeping, and I felt anxious about the surgery.

There is a reason hospitals make you sign consent forms. You aren't so much taking your health and life into your own hands as you are putting them in the hands of others. I know that surgery is dangerous, that getting an anaesthetic is dangerous. I know mistakes happen. I know you can die in hospitals. These thoughts flooded my mind in the middle of the night when pain wouldn't let me sleep and I was feeling scared and alone.

One month into the wait, I had my pre-op appointment. They do these things every day. I and about a dozen other orthopaedic patients showed up at Toronto Western for

8:30 a.m. The more coffee addicted among us had arrived even earlier to grab another cup before the day got fully under way. The other patients were a curious mix: some were there for their second or even third replacement of hips and knees, but most were like me, getting a first joint replacement. I had blood and X-rays taken, bacterial swabs done, and health records updated. I met physical therapists and ward nurses. I was taken through what was going to happen and what to expect both on the day of the surgery and in the first few days afterward. We were given detailed and repeated instructions on how to bathe before the day of surgery. Toronto Western, like most hospitals, is deeply concerned about the spread of methicillin-resistant *Staphylococcus aureus* (MRSA), an antibiotic-resistant staph bacteria, and takes numerous measures to counteract the possibility of a hospital infection or epidemic. It was the closest I have ever been to a dress rehearsal for a medical procedure, and it reassured me.

But my favourite encounter of the day was with the anesthesiologist, who discussed with me the options available for the operation. I can barely tolerate the idea, let alone the experience, of a general anaesthetic. It is an eerie, inexplicable feeling that I have endured too many times. At the back of my mind, since my first conversation with Dr. Syed, the only real trepidation had to do with the reality of going under one more time. Every anaesthetic carries risks, and I believe I have been forced into this gamble too many times. When the anesthesiologist explained that general anaesthetics were no longer used for hip surgeries and that the norm now was a spinal block and a range of sedatives, I experienced a wave of relief. With that worry out of the way, my curiosity kicked in and I started asking every question I could about how spinal blocks work, what levels of sedation were available and whether I could choose to be awake during the surgery. He was a bit taken aback at the idea that a patient might want to be awake, but suggested I discuss that with the anesthesiologist on duty that day.

Spinal blocks are pretty simple in conception. They are the equivalent of that old question: if a tree falls in the forest and there is no one around, does it make a sound? We feel pain because nerve receptors register shocks, insults and injuries and send the signals to the brain. In response, we tend to experience the appropriate level and type of pain. In surgery, the shock and attack are extreme and acute, but if you can stop the nerves from telling the brain what is going on, then for all intents and purposes, and for as long as you can block the signals, you aren't experiencing pain. So the anesthesiologist injects a needle through the lower back into the spinal space, which is filled with cerebral spinal fluid and encases the brain and the spinal cord. Local anaesthetics and other medications are injected, and communication between the lower body and the brain is severed. A key problem is that eventually the spinal block wears off, somewhere between one and four hours after the end of the procedure, and then the nerves and pain receptors go into overdrive, catching the brain up on what has been going on. When I was talking with the anesthesiologist at my pre-op session, I was so pleased that there would be no general anaesthetic that I didn't give much thought to what might happen after the surgery.

The one discordant note during the whole day came when I asked which rehabilitation hospital I would be sent to after being discharged from Toronto Western. Dr. Syed had been clear with Debi and me that, given the relatively extreme nature of my surgery, I would need a period of time in rehab before I could go home. The staff running the pre-op session said that as far as they could see, I was scheduled to be sent home when I was finished surgery, not to rehab. They acknowledged that Dr. Syed might have other plans.

There was just a month to go.

25

SURGERY

For much of the week of August 19, 2012, I did what I love to do: sit on our front porch, drink coffee, read, nod to or talk with our neighbours, and engage with strangers as they stop and stare in awe at Debi's incredible garden. Between trying to remember the name of a particular flower or where I was in the book I was attempting to finish, I would often find my mind obsessing about the surgery that Thursday.

I also spent the week forcing myself to walk. On days when Debi wasn't teaching, we would go to Home Smith Park and she'd walk a couple of miles and I'd walk a bit more than a mile. It hurt, some days more than others, but it was a pattern I was used to and it allowed me to engage in a form of walking meditation. I also used it as a tease: just imagine, I thought, in a few months, walking this route will be much easier and I'll be able to do it with no pain.

The night before the surgery, I had to undertake a harsh cleanse and abstain from eating. The cleanse, forcing myself to drink a couple of litres of truly horrendous purgative, is something I have never grown used to, though it is much preferable to the pre-surgery enemas I endured as a child. Both the cleanse and the enema are awkward and debilitating, but the enema has the added sting of the patient being denied any and all privacy and dignity. The abstention from food is not a big deal, but I do love my coffee. The day of my surgery, scheduled for 1:00 p.m., I was allowed to have black coffee early in the morning, a concession I much appreciated.

I didn't sleep much and was up early, taking advantage of the permission to have a coffee, when the hospital called and asked if we could move the surgery up. I said yes, let's get it over with. Checking in for surgery has changed over the years, and I was intrigued that nowadays I had to find my own way to the operating theatre pre-op area, where I was given a set of gowns by a very outgoing nurse along with clear directions on dressing for surgery. She came back into the room a few minutes later, looked at me and said, "So, sir, what day is it?"

"Thursday," I said.

"And why are you here at the hospital?" she said.

"I am having surgery."

"And what's your name?"

"Peter Kavanagh, and why are you asking me all these truly banal questions?"

"I am just checking your awareness level and your state of mind."

"Trust me, my awareness level is fine and my state of mind is good."

"Then is there another explanation for how you managed to put on those gowns completely backwards to the way I explained to you?"

I looked at myself and realized I had blown it completely. She laughed, I changed, and then she did a basic physical. She advised me that it was regular procedure to ask a patient repeatedly who they were, their date of birth, the procedure they were undergoing and what day it was. It was all part of making sure that the patient was fully aware of what was going on and, just as important, making sure that the medical staff were dealing with the right patient and performing the right procedure.

After about two hours in the pre-op area, having been given a slight sedative, I said goodbye to Debi and walked with a nurse to the operating room. Hospitals are filled with long corridors that stretch past doors behind which all kinds of mysterious things are going on. The walk to the OR as a patient is one of the strangest walks a human being can do. Despite the presence of my nurse companion, I felt very alone, deeply anxious and scared.

The operating room was cold, and within minutes I was shivering. Everyone there—nurses, interns, residents, surgeons and technicians—wore surgical gowns, and the neatest footwear: shoes, sneakers, running shoes of all colours and shapes, bold and brilliant. In an environment where all the clothes were the same, the operating team were displaying their personalities through their shoes. I was mesmerized by the shoe show as an anesthesiologist asked me to lean over a bar face first. He administered the spinal block, someone else brushed my lower body with an antiseptic wash, and a third person smeared ink on my left hip. Every few minutes someone asked me my name and why I was there and what day it was. Then I went under.

My recollections of the surgery itself are pretty sketchy. I was very cold, there were noises and the clink and clank of metal instruments hitting metal and porcelain trays. The light was extreme, bright and seemingly everywhere. There are odd smells in an operating room: chemical and body odours, iodine, disinfectants—that weird mix of olfactory sensations that we call medicinal. There was, as promised, no general anaesthetic, but the sedatives were powerful enough to put me to sleep, especially after the anesthesiologist and I had a bit of a set-to early on in the surgery.

"How are you doing?" the anesthesiologist asked.

"My arm is cold," I said.

"Hold on a second. How's that feel?"

"Now it is hot."

"It happens. The mix of drugs we use has different effects on different people, so we adjust the mix. Sometimes there's cold, sometimes there's hot, so it's all about finding the balance."

"Do you actually have double-blind clinical trials that prove this?" I asked.

"What?" the anesthesiologist said.

"I said, do you have clinical trials that back this up?"

"I think someone needs a nap," the anesthesiologist said.

Some time passed, and the next thing I heard was a voice I recognized as belonging to Dr. Syed.

"We are almost done," he said.

"Whoever said that must have children," I said.

"What? What do you mean?" he said.

"Almost done is like almost there. It has no meaning. I need reference points for that. How long has the surgery been going on? Are we three-quarters of the way through a four-hour operation or halfway through a one-hour operation?"

"There's a bit too much talking going on here," the surgeon said.

I fell asleep once again.

I woke again as I was being wheeled out of the operating room to recovery. I slowly started to make sense of my surroundings and realized that I had survived surgery once more. Nurses kept coming over to take my pulse and ask my name and why I was there. After about an hour I was wheeled to the orthopaedic ward on the ninth floor. All the while, I was feeling groggy but fine.

Dr. Syed came to my room to talk. He told Debi and me that the surgery had gone well and he had been able to fix the hip. He went on to say that he had been able to make my legs what they would have been like when I was a baby.

For a moment we were confused. He explained that in

addition to building me a new hip, he had lengthened my left leg such that it was now the same length as my right, something that had previously been true for only a brief time, more than five decades earlier. His quick explanation was that after constructing a hip socket and ball out of titanium, he'd created some artificial bone and screwed it into the femur, pushing the newly lengthened bones down in the skin of the leg so as to line my two legs up and make my whole lower body symmetrical.

I just stared at him, stared down at my legs, and then looked over at Debi and Jane, completely at a loss for words. I could tell by the looks on their faces that Debi and Jane were as bewildered as I was. I didn't know what to say. I started babbling about how none of my shoes, with their built-up heels, would work anymore. Dr. Syed smiled and said he thought having to buy all new shoes was a pretty small price to pay for having two legs that were the same length.

While we were trying to absorb all that Dr. Syed had told us, the spinal block wore off.

I am not a fan of painkillers, especially morphine. I had it during my "not colon cancer" surgery and I could not abide the hallucinations and delirium. Under morphine, my sense of body vanishes and my mind wheels and adopts the style, mania and frenzy of Road Runner cartoons. I feel dissociated and out of control. So I'd made it known before the surgery that I did not want morphine. The difficulty for the medical personnel was that morphine is very effective and the alternatives are less so. So for the first few hours the nurses and I were in a struggle to somehow get ahead of the pain such that I could relax and sleep. In the pre-op materials that I had been given, there were numerous tips on how to manage pain without drugs or along with drugs, suggestions such as the use of camomile teas and meditation. I was drinking the tea and meditating, but I was losing the battle. I was nearly hysterical with the pain. At one point it was so bad I believed it would never end, and that idea was so unbearable that I burst into tears. Of course eventually the drugs did click in, the pain became manageable, and within a few days the acute post-operative pain was pretty much gone. What no one had warned me about was that I would then have to deal with a very different type of pain.

One analogy for our nervous system is a telephone system connecting different parts of the body and the brain—a two-way communications device. The nerves are the equivalent of wires connecting various regions and organs of the body with head office, and the pathways can be damaged by "pressure, stretching or cutting."

As Dr. Syed explained to me, one of the consequences of pushing the leg down, stretching the skin and muscle and extending the bone, is a form of "neural implosion." All of the nerves from mid-thigh down to the tips of my toes went dark. No messages were being sent, and none were there to be retrieved. This alarmed me, but Dr. Syed was very calm as he explained the connection between the leg lengthening and the silent nerves, and his equanimity somehow reassured me.

Within twenty-four hours, I began experiencing the oddest array of sensations and symptoms in my left leg: cramps, feelings of deep burning and bitter cold, tingling and twinges and varieties of pins and needles and total numbness. These "impressions" came in rapid succession and not in any particular or regular pattern. Dr. Syed was quite pleased to hear this, and said it meant the nerves were rebuilding themselves. The odd sensations were the equivalent of a nerve firing a signal to the brain and the brain taking a stab at interpreting what the nerve was trying to say. So a nerve sends a signal and the brain thinks, "Wow . . . that's cold . . . no, wait, that's hot, no, wrong again, that signal is really a spasm." And on and on this goes. The one thing Dr. Syed and I agreed on was that where there is sensation, there are living nerves, and living nerves engaged in the process of repairing themselves is a good thing and much preferable to any and all alternatives. The difficulty was that nerves take a long time to repair themselves. Nerves regenerate at about one millimetre a day, so it can take a while for a whole leg to repair itself.

The day after surgery, a status report read, "Still groggy, still experiencing pain, nerve damage and rebuilding." Some folks from physiotherapy showed up to get me out of bed and see how I might do at walking, giving me a glimpse of what the next few months were going to be like. The standard operating procedure after hip surgery is that the patient is standing the next day and beginning initial walking, and by the third or fourth day is being discharged from the hospital to go home. Debi and I were still getting mixed signals, with Dr. Syed saying he believed I should and would be going to a rehabilitation hospital while the nurses and rehabilitation staff kept insisting that I was going to be discharged in a couple of days according to the normal routine.

Getting out of bed and trying to walk, even with a chest-high walker, was not a grand success. Two men from physiotherapy helped me get out of bed and stand, relatively speaking. I was told not to put any real pressure on my left leg and foot but, despite that, I should try to walk using the walker, my good upper-body strength and my strong right leg. My brain was fuzzy and tired, my body still feeling the aftershocks of surgery, my left leg cramping and experiencing pins and needles, but most of all my left leg felt like a piece of wood. I couldn't move it. I thought, if this is what walking post-surgery is going to be like, then my quality of life has gone seriously downhill. I told one of the physiotherapists that this effort at walking felt weird and awkward and was wearing me out. They told me to keep moving a little bit longer. When I got back into bed, I fell into a deep sleep.

When I woke up, I started to think through that disastrous first attempt at walking. I realized there were three different problems that were making walking difficult.

The first problem was the injunction from Dr. Syed against putting any real weight on my left leg for at least the first three months after surgery. The way it was explained to me was that I could put some weight and pressure on the left leg, but only the amount that would be involved in putting my toes on a raw egg without breaking the shell. How would anyone know how much weight that is?

The second problem was that the muscles in my left leg weren't really functioning at that moment. Nerves control muscles, but there were no truly functioning nerves in my leg, and the muscles in that leg had never been top-notch anyway.

The third difficulty I had with that first walk was something that had me truly perplexed: I didn't know where my left foot actually was.

26

REHAB

Our pop culture is filled with references to rehab. Amy Winehouse became famous for refusing to go, Lindsay Lohan spent seemingly endless hours in court arguing about rehab and sentencing provisions regarding her time there, movies and television series dealing with the Iraq and Afghan wars invariably have scenes built around wounded soldiers undergoing rehab. Rehab has become a ubiquitous culture icon that few have actually had to wrestle with.

Rehabilitation hospitals themselves aren't a new idea. Many such facilities in North America have their origins in 1919, as communities struggled to cope with the long-term consequences of World War I, a devastating war in terms of fatalities, and arguably even more so for its survivors who suffered significant physical and mental damage. That's when the Toronto Rehabilitation Centre opened, with a very specific mandate to address the needs of veterans.

The concept of physical rehabilitation is as old as Hippocrates but first emerged as a "real" discipline in 1813 with the growth of orthopaedics as a separate branch of medicine. The idea that you could "fix" the human body, as opposed to "curing" it of disease, generated a whole slew of ancillary fields and expertise. If you were going to attempt remedies of smashed, deformed and inadequate limbs, then you needed to develop the means and techniques to make it possible to use these repaired limbs and approximations of limbs in ways that at least resembled the normal use of a leg or an arm. If you have a prosthetic leg, you need to be able to walk with it. If you have an artificial hand, you need to be able to hold things with it. While we like to think that walking and grasping are normal and innate actions, the reality is that every time you change the basic conditions, there is new learning to be done. And most of us need help learning.

Hospitals are institutions, and they have fiefdoms and jurisdictional battles. Toronto Western is no different. For the first few days after my surgery, I kept running into what was clearly a long-simmering dispute between surgeons and physiotherapists over who made the decisions about rehab. After my first attempt at standing and moving, Debi and I were convinced that going directly from the hospital to home was going to be very difficult, and Dr. Syed agreed. We next raised it with the physiotherapy coordinator, and she told us that a decision had yet to be made. We said Dr. Syed had told us otherwise, and she sharply informed us that surgeons didn't decide who went to rehab, physiotherapists did, and she would get back to us. It was the same dispute, in updated language, that Sister Kenny and the medical profession had had sixty years earlier, in the darkest days of the polio epidemic.

Variations on the conversations involving Dr. Syed and the physiotherapy coordinator happened a few times during the first two days after my surgery. I was less groggy and experiencing the most incredible series of spasms and nerve shocks throughout my leg. My mental state was a weird combination of excitement, anxiety, pain and serenity. But my key concern was getting the rehab I needed.

Three days in, it was announced that the next morning I was going to be moved to Hillcrest Rehab Hospital. Hillcrest was opened in the 1880s as a long-term care facility and morphed into a rehabilitation facility in the 1970s. By the time I arrived in 2012, it was on the verge of becoming part of a massive new rehab facility in the downtown core. There were tile floors and antibacterial soap hand dispensers everywhere. The staff was what you would find in any ordinary hospital, but there was the additional layer of physiatrists (doctors trained in rehabilitation medicine), physiotherapists and occupational therapists. The other key differences between ordinary hospitals and rehab hospitals are the presence of gyms and exercise rooms as well as the seeming commitment to keep the patient for the optimal amount of time so that discharge doesn't mean setback.

Getting from Toronto Western to Hillcrest involved a slow drive up Bathurst Street in an ambulance. Strapped into a gurney, flat on my back and staring out the rear-door windows, I was momentarily transported back to Fredericton, twelve years old and being taken home in a body cast. I knew it was best that I go to rehab before heading home, but I really had no idea how long I would be in Hillcrest. It was a funny, sad-achy feeling, being fifty-nine years old and wondering how I ended up being twelve all over again.

After I checked in, two young women, one a physiotherapist and the other an occupational therapist, popped into my room to do an assessment. Physiotherapists, or PTs, are fixated on trying to get the body working correctly, or as correctly as possible, while occupational therapists, or OTs, focus on helping with life hacks, the workarounds that allow the patient to approximate a normal life, while working toward something more akin to what daily life is about to become. So the PT designs exercises aimed at reactivating muscles and strengthening fundamental processes and sequences, while the OT makes sure the patient can dress, take a shower or cook without always requiring the assistance of another. Being shown how to put on my pants might seem pretty small-scale, but given that I hadn't yet figured out how to do it without leaning over or bending my legs or putting weight on my left leg, it was a major accomplishment. Much of what my OT showed me seemed trivial but was truly significant. There are tools available: grabbers, sock guides, long brushes for showers and a number of other devices that make navigating the various rooms of the house easier. What I learned from the OT at Hillcrest dramatically increased the quality of my recuperation. It reinforced for me the idea that all technologies are adaptive. Until forced, we never pay attention to how much we all rely on tools and machines to get us through our day. The grabber I used to pick things up off the floor only seems funny until you are forbidden to bend at the waist. Attitude adjustment is also at the heart of OT: fixating on and attending to what you are doing at the moment. Occupational therapy is really a form of mindfulness.

Physiotherapy is a different ball game altogether, maybe even the tougher of the two disciplines. The big difference I found between OT and PT is that physiotherapy is for the most part an internal regimen. Sure, there are equipment and tools, but physiotherapy really depends on what you are made of and what you can summon up. Occupational therapy gives you the tools to get your shoes on and tied; physiotherapy demands that you move and exercise.

Hillcrest was an intriguing mix of old and young, though it definitely skewed old. At fifty-nine, I was considered by many of the other patients and the staff to be one of the "youngsters" in the facility. While I was there, the range of the other patients and their problems was broad: a lot of people doing rehab after knee or hip surgery, some recovering from strokes, victims of serious car crashes. My routines were pretty much the norm: in the morning I went to the gym, in the afternoon I walked up and down corridors, in between I rested and took painkillers. The doctors and the nurses emphasized that my body needed to heal and that meant I had to find a balance between exercise, rest and painkillers.

When I arrived in the exercise room the morning after checking into Hillcrest, I chatted with my new physio-therapist about my surgery, my medical history and my walking problems in the past. Then I tried some simple exercises while lying on a raised bed: spreading my legs and bringing them back together in snow-angel fashion, lifting my leg and straightening my knee. While I was doing these basic moves, my therapist just watched me. She asked me to stop and lie flat on my back. She had me close my eyes and she moved my legs and the lower part of my body to the side. She asked me to keep my eyes closed and to move my legs and lower body to the point where I believed my body to be straight. I remember thinking this was a very pecu-liar request, but I complied. When I said I thought I was straight, she told me to keep my eyes closed and she moved my legs and asked me to describe if my body was now straight or at an angle. I told her I thought I was at a signifi-cant angle. She told me to open my eyes and look down. I was lying perfectly straight.

She also had me stand in front of a floor-to-ceiling mirror and close my eyes and move so that I was standing straight. When I had done so and opened my eyes, I realized how significant a tilt I had. I'd always joked that I was a ter-rible judge of whether things on a wall were straight because I spent my life at an angle. That morning, I learned it wasn't really a joke.

Physiotherapy is an odd combination of science, on-the-spot innovation, clinical psychology and motivational speaking. There was one PT at Hillcrest by the name of Lucky—his actual name. He looked like a football player, seemed as fit as a US Marine, and had a deep, mellifluous Caribbean accent. He clearly loved his job and was an intensely caring presence. He'd chant out phrases designed to make me laugh even while I sweated the most agonizing movement. "Don't look at the ground as you walk, there's no money on the ground, I already found it, look straight ahead as you walk." "Don't rush through your exercises, this isn't boot camp, if this was boot camp, we'd all be dead. Take your time, do them right." I remember one time in particular, when he was trying to encourage an older Greek woman who was recovering from hip surgery. She was feeling low and in pain and just wanted to go back to her room, and he wanted her to try to do the exercises for the day. She whined, sobbed and asked to be allowed to go to her room, and he agreed she could go after she did some knee bends. It was a standoff. She looked away and muttered in another language. He spun around, snapped out a sentence in the same language and then said in English, "Don't swear at me in Greek. Do the knee bends and you can go back to your room." She looked stunned, then proceeded to do the knee bends as well as the rest of the exercises on the list. Later on, I said that I was impressed he knew Greek. He said he didn't, just a few words from vacationing in Greece, but he figured she had been cursing and thought he could put the fear of God into her. He smiled and said he'd learned to do it with a few languages and it worked.

It was at Hillcrest that I first began piecing together the problem of my out-of-place foot. Discovering, that first time I tried walking after surgery, that I didn't actually have a firm sense of where my left foot was continued to bother me. I had assumed the confusion arose from a combination of grogginess and painkillers. But at Hillcrest, when I was much better rested and the drugs were not nearly as potent, the problem of the out-of-place foot continued. I am normally not conscious of where the various parts of my body are at any particular moment; most of us aren't. I count on my subconscious mind to know the positioning of my body to the degree necessary for me to move about without stumbling and tripping over myself. Post-surgery, though, I was stumbling, tripping and shoving my foot into obstacles such as table legs and door jambs as if my brain was unaware that my foot was even there. The mind usually has a three-dimensional sense of the space the body is occupying in the world, but it seemed that might not be the case for me anymore.

A couple of days after I checked into Hillcrest, one of the doctors dropped into my room to talk.

"I've been reading your file," he said. "It's very interesting. Your operation was about as far as one can get from a routine hip operation. Mind if I take a look at your leg?"

"Go ahead," I said. "I want to ask you about my sense of where my foot is. It's like I don't know where my foot is without looking at it."

"Yeah, the phantom limb problem with a twist," he said. "You know about the phantom limb phenomenon, where the brain thinks an arm or a leg is still there even though it's been amputated?"

"Yeah, but I'm not sure how that fits."

"Sometimes the brain gets confused. For five decades your brain has thought your leg was in one place and now it's in another place. You and your brain have to learn where the new location of your leg is. It's the type of thing you have to expect when you have surgery like this, surgery that's about as far from a routine hip operation as you can get."

"That's twice you've described my operation as about as far from a routine operation as you can get. Should that worry me?"

The doctor paused slightly and then said, "No. But you have to admit it is interesting."

Newtonian physics postulates that a body in motion tends to stay in motion and a body at rest tends to stay at rest. Physiotherapists need to get patients moving, exercising damaged muscles and joints so that they can repair themselves. The patient's natural tendency is to avoid pain and fatigue, which are associated with exercise and exertion. The patient and the PT are on the same page: both want the patient out of the hospital free of constraints and living as normal a life as possible. The PT knows from experience what this is going to take, while the patient only knows himself and is intent on taking the path of least resistance. Paradoxically, sometimes the PT has to slow a patient down, bring them a reality check about what they can and cannot do. As with many of the things a PT does, it is a tricky balance.

For several weeks, my routine was the same. I woke early, ate, took some painkillers, went down to physiotherapy, wore myself out, returned to my room, slept, ate again, walked the halls, exercised, ate again, slept and began again. The exercises were very simple and very hard. Stand up at parallel bars and try to do five slight knee bends; sit in a chair and hold your knees together with your hands and try to push the knees apart; while lying down, try to move your legs apart and bring them together again. As simple as the exercises were, the pain they could cause was extreme. I would go back to my room after a half-hour in the exercise room and lie down on my bed exhausted. My leg would be clenching up, throbbing, burning, alternating numbness with tingles, and my biggest priority was trying to get to sleep and put it all aside for a few hours.

What I could not shake was a constant sense of déjà vu that animated every physiotherapy session. I had done all of this when I was a toddler, and again when I was a teen. The exercise room, crutches, wheelchairs, parallel bars, thick elastic bands, pulleys, weights, mock stairs, heating pads and ice packs were all so familiar. The exhortations, hints, suggestions and admonitions of the physiotherapists were both new and old. I hadn't heard these particular physiotherapists tell me how to flex a muscle or bend a leg before, but I knew their type. Scenes from previous efforts kept competing with the present. But just as I had to focus on how to lift *this* knee, I had to focus on *this* experience *now*, another exercise in mindfulness. What was important was what I was doing right and wrong *today*, not what I had failed at decades earlier. At night, when I reviewed how the day had gone—what I had done well, what surprised me, what disappointed me and what I should concentrate on tomorrow—sometimes what bewildered me most was how much time I had spent reliving old efforts instead of being present in these new ones.

My preoccupation with the past wasn't confined to the physiotherapy sessions. Hospital rooms everywhere are pretty much alike: same basic structure, construction materials and furniture. During the rest periods of the day, on my bed in my room, I would slip into memories of previous hospital stays. At any given moment, staring out the window down Bathurst Street, I would find myself thirteen again and looking out a hospital window at the Saint John River in Fredericton, New Brunswick, or nine and trying not to cry in the loneliness of the Children's Hospital in Calgary. Late at night, after evening medication had been administered, I would lie on my bed and stare at the acoustic tiles in the ceiling and try to calculate how many hours of my life I had spent doing just that.

On reflection, it seems so quotidian, and it was: I was fixated on conquering the day-to-day. It was remarkable how much joy the simple things evoked, like seven days after my surgery when I was able, using a walker, to shower on my own. It was a luxury, the memory of which still brings me a warm glow. Learning to walk again was slow and tedious, but mastering even these slight things thrilled me. The day I was able to slowly navigate my way out of the building using a wheelchair, to sit in an Adirondack chair and simply soak up the sun, all without the aid of a nurse or PT, gave me a real sense that I could do this. A week later, on the day I did it with crutches, it was that much better.

I learned during the three weeks after my surgery that when you are in rehab, willpower and determination are key. For a few days at Hillcrest I shared a room with a teenager who had been terribly smashed up in a car crash and was facing months and months of extreme pain and even more extreme hard work. He was a deflated individual with no obvious sense of determination, and his PT and nurses were hounding him all the time to move, exercise and take control, all to very little avail. He spent most of his time either playing video games on a laptop or reading sports magazines. He didn't talk much and seemed to have no sense of how his recovery was going to play out. During the same period, I would run into a guy in the gym who was in his early eighties. He had just undergone his seventh joint replacement and you couldn't keep him away from the parallel bars and artificial stairs they had scattered everywhere. He said to me one day, "I just can't wait to get home to play with the grandkids." Motivation matters, determination matters, attitude matters. Assuming the physical has been handled relatively well and that there are no structural or biological problems, the mental state is the difference between mastering this learning-to-walk thing or not.

But this concentration on conquering the day-to-day had a downside: my routine became a slog. That first rush of joy at getting the hang of something new or relearning some old activity gave way to the realization that from here on it was all about maintaining momentum, keeping to a schedule. After three weeks, my time at Hillcrest was clearly, in my mind at least, coming to an end. I believed I had learned what they had to teach me. I had the basic exercises down. I had absorbed the lessons of the OTs and had learned how to cope when no one else was around. I had learned the things I needed to do in order to go home. My being home would make things easier for Debi and Jane, as they wouldn't have to disrupt their routines to come and see me at the hospital, and of course it would be much easier on me. I was ready to leave.

My PTs agreed that it might be time for me to go, but they explained that the one stumbling block was that I needed a physiotherapy plan in place before I could be discharged. I had anticipated this and had made arrangements to go to a neighbourhood physiotherapy centre, Pivot Sport Medicine. I had used them before for massages, they had a great reputation, and I really liked the staff. The only possible hitch in my mind was that Pivot was on the second floor of a building, with twenty-eight steps from the sidewalk to the clinic entrance, and there was no elevator. I was on crutches and not allowed to put weight on my left leg. When I explained the Pivot arrangement to the PTs, they were adamant that this clinic was not an option, that I needed some other plan.

I was disappointed by their response, angry even, and told them so.

I fumed overnight, convinced that all these otherwise helpful individuals were being bureaucratically obstinate on this one point. The next day I asked if the issue was that climbing twenty-eight steps would wear me out or that the climb would be harmful to the healing of my hip and leg. It was the wearing me out that they were concerned with. They insisted that twenty-eight steps is a lot on crutches and especially just after surgery. I was not a novice with crutches and suggested that if I could demonstrate that I could do twenty-eight steps, then they should let me go home. They said sure. I could tell by their grins that they were pretty confident how this would go. Using an inner stairwell, I went up and down two flights of stairs. Their grins changed to true smiles and they told me I could go home.

Almost four weeks after my surgery, Debi picked me up at Hillcrest. Everything about healing the body is complicated. I had to back up and sit sideways on a special cushion atop the passenger seat in the front of the car. I had to lift my legs—but not too high—and swing around until I was facing forward. Then, of course, I had to somehow position my crutches so that they were nearby but not blocking the driver. And if I thought I was quickly getting better, the twenty-minute drive home showed me otherwise. It had been weeks since I had sat anywhere near the way you sit in a car, and my legs felt confined in that position. The cramping and tingling in my left leg seemed to intensify, and all together these various discomforts almost made me scream.

Then there was a whole new set of issues at home. The entrance to our house from the driveway is through a basement door next to the garage. From there I had to go up twelve steps to the kitchen, then down a hallway and up another fifteen steps to our bedroom. By the time I had made it to the bedroom, a little under an hour after we had left Hillcrest, I was completely exhausted. As I settled into my own bed for the first time in more than a month, I realized just how long this whole process was going to be.

27

TWENTY-EIGHT STEPS UP, TWENTY-EIGHT STEPS DOWN

Navigating the twenty-eight steps into Pivot Sport Medicine in October, not quite two months after my surgery, was difficult, partly because it was first thing in the morning and my leg muscles weren't clicking in, partly because I hadn't had enough coffee, and, in hindsight, mostly because the physical reality of the stair-climbing routine had started to sink in.

I met with Vaiva Underys. She has her master's degree in clinical science in manipulative therapy from the University of Western Ontario and is a runner. She asked a lot of smart questions and listened carefully to everything I said. We hit it off almost immediately. She was fascinated by my surgery, and with what the surgeon was attempting with my leg. She had me walk about a bit on the crutches and then had me move my leg as best I could. She explained that the first big problem was that there was not much we could do until the restriction on placing weight on my leg was lifted. She watched me do the exercises I had learned at Hillcrest, gave me a few tips on technique and made some suggestions about other exercises I could try at home.

For the next few weeks, until late November 2012, my day-to-day life was dull and tiring, largely consisting of exercises, moving about with crutches, resting and reading. The leg raises, leg lifts and muscle strengthening became easier, but it was hard for me to see how this all connected with actual walking.

Every Monday, Dr. Syed has clinic hours at Toronto Western, and on the last Monday in November, three months after the surgery, he and I met up. Clinic appointments are time-consuming, Dr. Syed is always running late, and the waiting room is usually filled with people with a range of casts, crutches and canes. I went for X-rays and waited for hours with Debi. When we were finally called into an exam room, everybody was all smiles. Dr. Syed told me that the X-rays looked great, the leg and hip were healing nicely, and the restriction against putting weight on the leg was lifted. I was relieved that the recovery was going as planned. I was also slightly apprehensive. Up until now, learning to walk had been more theoretical than anything else. Now it would get real, and if my past experiences were anything to go by, getting real is synonymous with being difficult.

The next day, I met with Vaiva and we started work in earnest. Being able to put weight on the leg meant real exercises. Weight bearing means building up muscle and capacity. Resistance exercises that I had been doing had been protecting the leg from further deterioration, but I knew that the real work would come with relearning how to use the leg the way the leg was supposed to be used. Before we could really get going on this part of my recovery, though, I needed to solve the problem of my brace.

28

A NEW BRACE

For thirty-four years—the first sixteen and the last eighteen—I have worn a brace on my left leg. The twenty-five years in between glow in my memory with happiness and unfettered joy. A moment's reflection dispels that rose-coloured perception and leaves me with many unanswerable what-ifs. If I had worn a brace for those twenty-five in-between years, would my walking today be better, easier, more manageable and more normal? Would wearing a brace have made any difference to my post-operative condition? Would a consistent life of wearing a brace have created a different personality, a different me? Would I be an individual who has no esteem issues about my walking? How do I answer these questions without shaking my head, smirking or pouring another grappa? The answer is I can't, and I don't. I accept that for part of my sixty years and counting, I didn't wear a brace. But my brace and I are, for good or for ill, one.

The thing I never struggled with or devoted any real thought to in all those years of wearing a brace and not wearing one were the really difficult questions about brace design, brace utility and brace functionality. What was this thing wrapped around my leg, how did it work, and were all braces created equal?

Leg braces come in four main types: Ankle-Foot (AFO), Knee-Ankle-Foot (KAFO), Hip-Knee-Ankle-Foot (HKAFO) and Thoracolumbarsacral Orthosis (TLSO). The difference is what part of the body needs support and whether the key issue is weight transfer, muscle and bone support or gait alignment. The key factors in determining how to build the brace include gait, balance, posture and the location of paralyzed muscles.

During childhood and into my teens, my braces were steel with leather cuffs and straps fixed into the built-up heel of a heavy shoe. In the mid-nineties, after I had broken my foot one too many times, my brace was hard moulded plastic with Velcro straps at the ankle and the knee, and it slipped inside shoes with a built-up heel. After my surgery and the lengthening of my leg, I really needed a new style of brace, one that was more flexible than rigid plastic and provided support instead of height. I no longer needed to artificially even out my body, but I did need something that would give my newly lengthened leg some critical support.

A new brace became crucial when I started doing physiotherapy at Pivot Sport Medicine. The pre-surgery brace cupped my foot from below and ran up the back of my left leg, and was fastened right above the ankle and below the knee. Once I had it on, I would slide the brace-encased foot into a built-up shoe. The two built-up pieces helped bridge the distance between my foot and the ground and kept my leg rigid. After my surgery, there was no physical distance between my foot and the ground, but there was theoretical distance. My mind's perception of where my foot was, my odd lifelong posture of leaning to the right, and the way I habitually held my leg and foot meant there was a distance that needed to be overcome through exercise, physiotherapy and habit.

All the shoes I owned had built-up heels and required that I wear my built-up brace. My surgeon thought I should be able to go without a brace. My physiotherapist figured that, while with time my leg would be flexible enough to rest on the ground without a brace, I would still need one given that I had always lacked the ability to lift my left foot. My orthotist refused to make me a less built-up brace, let alone a flat brace, because my foot didn't touch the ground when I stood. It was a circular reasoning that had me completely baffled. How was I going to do this? How was I going to get to the stage of walking normally, without a built-up shoe and brace, if I couldn't break the cycle of needing to wear a built-up brace and shoe? Of the three professionals—the physiotherapist, the orthotist and the surgeon—who was actually the person to make the decision?

Vaiva, my physiotherapist, ended the standoff. She suggested that I ask my doctor for a prescription for a new brace that worked as an AFO for the purposes of lifting the foot and strengthening the muscles and leg. With the new brace and the right exercises and diligence, my foot would touch the ground. More excitingly, with a new brace I could get shoes that had no built-up heel. I took her suggestion to my surgeon and, as was always the case on these issues, he simply wanted to know what my physiotherapist thought. When I explained her reasoning, he wrote a prescription and I walked out of the hospital and across the street to a Walking Mobility Clinic, a chain that specializes in footwear, braces, assistive technologies and other services.

The pedorthist went through the history of the moulded plastic brace I was using and the surgery I had had, and asked about my goal. She thought for a while and suggested that the brace I had been wearing was the exact opposite of the type of brace I should now be wearing. Before my surgery I needed to protect a weakened leg that functioned poorly for a variety of reasons. Now I was trying to make a "rebuilt leg" function as normally as possible, so I needed a brace that would allow my muscles to strengthen, my tendons to lengthen and my leg to receive and give feedback as I grew more confident and my walking improved. I didn't need a piece of plastic that encased my leg and kept it rigid, but something that supported my leg and allowed it to flex.

That's how I ended up wearing Kevlar on my leg. My brace is light—much lighter than the plastic brace—and has a thin plate beneath my foot and an equally thin bar that runs up the front left side of my left leg. It has Velcro fasteners at the ankle and just below the knee. It allows my foot to lift, it makes my gait potentially more normal, and it makes the leg feel more dynamic and reactive. This brace got me closer to the feeling I had when I wasn't wearing a brace at all. Most importantly, my Kevlar brace meant I could now plunge into physiotherapy.

29

BUILDING A
WORKING LEG

Once I could put weight on my leg, three months after surgery, I started doing the exercises that involved me using my left leg to pull and push weights, learning to shift my body weight off my dominant right leg and onto my weaker left leg. It was at times a bewildering mix of exercise, sequence and purpose, and it was especially confusing to know which exercises I was supposed to do first.

Physio always begins with my left foot on a pivot board and Vaiva forcing the foot up and down, getting a feel for how flexible it is that day. In the early days—and this is still true to some degree—I had no certain sense of how the foot was reacting or what the foot or leg was capable of. The nerves that were repairing themselves, the ones damaged in the neural implosion, were taking their time.

Then it is flexibility exercises, to increase the range of motion in my upper and lower leg muscles, and strengthening exercises, which are designed to increase the "bad" leg's ability to hold body weight while the "good" leg is off the ground—which, if you think about it, is about half the time when one is walking. Finally, there are balance exercises, designed to improve my ability to sway, stand, bend and flex, and in a sense to give me better judgment of what I am and am not capable of.

I do my physiotherapy with the help of heavy-duty stretch bands, rubber balls and mats, balance boards, mirrors, bars, weights, a treadmill and true human ingenuity. For the most part, Vaiva supplies the latter. When she asks me every time what's wrong or worrying me, she really means something like: "What are you trying to do while walking or using your leg that you cannot do, and which is causing you to worry?" Once, I told her that I couldn't cross my right leg over the top of my other leg. That's how I put a sock on my right foot, and not being able to cross that leg over meant I needed either a sock-putting-on device (there is one) or the assistance of another person; one way feels foolish and the other demeaning. Vaiva understood and came up with not a solution but an exercise. She pointed out that when crossing their legs, a human being needs to use the tendons at the back of the leg between the hip and the upper leg muscles. In my case, the tendons were not sufficiently stretched or flexible, and so I needed to do an exercise that strengthens and lengthens those tendons. On other occasions what has worried me most has been stepping up and down with my bad leg, or stopping the thigh muscle in my bad leg from freezing up such that it is painful to shift it even slightly, or—most problematically when walking without a cane, which I started attempting a few months after my first day at Pivot—making sure that I didn't have a hitch as I walked. In every case, after a bit of thought, Vaiva had a suggested exercise or routine that allowed me to tackle the problem on my own.

When I am not at Pivot, my daily routine begins with a walk up and down my block. In the early days after being allowed to put weight on the leg, I used crutches, but when I grew slightly more confident I switched to canes. When I return from my walk, I do a series of strange exercises. I put a tea towel on the floor, put my left foot flat on the tea towel, and slide it from side to side and back and forth, all the while keeping my foot flat. I sit on a chair with a large, tough rubber ball between my knees and bend up and down at the waist. I bring my knees together, wrap a large, heavy rubber band around them, and then force them apart as far as my strength and the band allow. I stand and hold a cane straight out to the side, stretching as far as I can to the left and then switching arms and repeating the movement, stretching as far as I can to the right. In both cases I try to stand up straight with my left foot flat on the floor and my left knee slightly bent. I sit on the edge of a bed and, with the aid of a towel wrapped around my upper thigh, try to lift my leg from the knee up. And after all these exercises are done, I walk some more.

When I walk, I focus on each and every piece of the process. I watch my right leg move from rest through swing to rest again, and then concentrate intently on each part of the same process with my left leg. While I move my left leg, it is important that the leg not swing out to the side, as if I am swinging it with my torso; instead, it needs to swing straight ahead through the action of my leg muscles. My natural inclination is to swing my leg, as that's partly how I compensated when it was shorter and much weaker than my right leg. Part of rewiring my walking is learning day by day where my foot is, where my leg is, and how to move the two in the way a foot and leg should move. I feel so foolish concentrating so hard on what is so simple in conception as I walk down my street, across a room in my house, through a shopping mall. But if I don't concentrate, if I don't focus, then I stumble or drag my foot or miss a step or send a jolt of pain through my leg. It is the same when standing still. My lifelong tendency is to list to one side, putting my weight on my right leg. If I don't pay attention, that is what I do. When I notice, I bring myself back to a balanced position. It is the physical equivalent of meditating and bringing your attention back to your breath. And just as in meditation, when I am supposed to not be judgmental but simply to note that my mind has wandered off and I need to return to my breath, so too when I find my body doing the things it has done for five decades, I shouldn't get angry or irritated or call myself names. But sometimes I do.

When I was feeling foolish or self-conscious, I was feeling frustrated. Nearly half a year after my surgery, I was still trying to get straight in my mind how long all of this was going to take. When I was prepping for surgery, one of the pieces of information provided was a rough timeline for how long it should take a person to recover from hip surgery and be walking normally again. In a best-case scenario, the average person could envision a three-to-six-month process. But as that curious doctor at Hillcrest noted repeatedly, I was as far from a routine case as one could get. So, for me, what was the best-case scenario?

30

THE ONGOING ISSUE
OF MIXED SIGNALS

I am by myself in the Toronto Western Hospital food court, waiting for an electromyography (EMG) test. That I am here alone is evidence that I am recovering. I navigated my way to the hospital using public transit and will navigate my way home the same way. I am using crutches and my walking is slow, ponderous and awkward, but I am out and about on my own. Despite this concrete proof of improvement, I am anxious.

An EMG test assesses the functioning of the nerves and muscles in the limbs. It is a diagnostic tool used to determine the existence and severity of nerve and muscle problems. The test is relatively simple: Electrodes that read the signals to and from muscles and along nerves are fixed to different parts of the leg. A technician uses a wand, which generates low-level electrical signals, to stimulate the nerve system at different points. The signals' strength or weakness is plotted on graphs and charts and read by specialists in the functioning of the neuroskeletal system, the various bits and pieces that make us moving, functioning beings.

I am having an EMG because of my ongoing concerns that the nerves in my leg and especially my foot haven't completely returned since the surgery and the neural implosion. I've been thinking that this slow neural recovery is making walking difficult because it seems to exacerbate my problem with truly sensing the location of my foot. It is nowhere near as severe as in those first few days after surgery, when my brain literally could not find my foot and was equally confused about my leg generally. There has been a return of sensation in my foot, which is now transmitting messages about the quality of the surface I am standing on and the temperature of its surroundings, but not to the degree that my right foot does or to the degree that I assume a normal foot does.

The hour-long test goes relatively smoothly and consists almost entirely of the steps described in a YouTube video I watched in advance, entitled "What to expect in an EMG test." I couldn't help but think while watching the video that this might truly be the best of times and the worst of times when it comes to the practice of medicine: the best of times because patients like me can bone up on all kinds of procedures and possible outcomes and thereby save the system time, and the worst of times because patients like me can bone up on all kinds of procedures and possible outcomes and thereby create all kinds of new and unexpected demands on the system and the professionals within it.

In December 2013, a few weeks after my EMG test, I see Dr. Syed to discuss it. The good news is that there is re-innervation in all the muscles in my leg, a relatively astounding phenomenon given my history and the odds we were all facing of seeing that happen. Dr. Syed seems surprised and pleased. Some days later, when I tell my physiotherapist about the report, she says she is both surprised and not. Vaiva explains that she has noticed the muscles in my leg growing and strengthening since I first started physio with her.

The bad news is that I have signs of peripheral neuropathy in my left foot. The impact of the neuropathy is partly a question of sensation and partly of balance and steadiness. We are learning more and more all the time about stance, balance and walking, and one of the things that is becoming clearer is that the systems our bodies use—senses, sensory input, nerve transmissions and the various levels of cranial calculations at the brain stem, cerebellum and cerebral cortex levels—to accomplish something as mundane and ordinary as standing straight, tall and even are agonizingly complex. What did this mean in the long term for my walking? No one had the answer or knew who might know.

31

THE TIMETABLE

No one has ever given me a firm timetable, a set of benchmarks or even an idea of the ultimate end state. When I first met with Dr. Syed in June 2012, he asked me what my goal was and I told him I wanted to spend a month in Vietnam walking about without a lot of pain. He nodded and said sure, that was possible. In every examination since the operation, I had raised my frustrations about the time that "getting back to normal" was taking. Of course, what I was really looking for was some clue as to when I'd be walking like other people, not like the old me with the different-length legs and awkward built-up shoes, which was the real normal I was looking for. Dr. Syed would nod and explain that one of the reasons I was a good patient was that I kept getting frustrated and working away, which pleased him. I would leave those encounters feeling pumped because I was "a good patient" and annoyed that my sense of how long this was going to take was no further advanced.

One day at Pivot, Vaiva introduced me to an intern doing her master's degree at Western and spending a few weeks in a physiotherapy practicum. After taking me through a series of regular exercises and having me walk a bit, Vaiva had me talk about my surgery. She then turned to the intern and said, "Can you believe it's only been a year since his surgery? Look at the progress he's made." The intern seemed impressed, but the only thought going through my mind was "It's been a year and I'm still here, still doing this."

In the months I have been going to physiotherapy, the one consistent thing I have noticed is that there seems to be no "typical" patient or end goal. There's the guy who wrecked his leg in a motorcycle accident, who is super-fit except for the one leg that was smashed to pieces. He's trying to get that leg back to the state where doing trampoline jumps and leaping on and off stairs is normal again. There is the woman in her fifties who injured her shoulder muscles and can't play her favourite sport of tennis until she can get those muscles back into ideal operating condition. There is the teenaged girl who is a gymnast and has injured her tendons and needs to get them back in shape before the next competition. There is the older man whose legs are in constant nerve pain; work is proving impossible and his doctor hopes some therapy might help get him back on the job. The walls of Pivot are festooned with posters signed by dancers, hockey players, musicians and whole orchestras thanking the staff for making it possible for them to continue doing what they love.

I am not a typical patient either. No one at Pivot has ever worked with a client who has had to learn to walk for a third time. My surgery and leg lengthening are new to Vaiva, so she doesn't have a timetable for me, any more than my surgeon does. The damage done to the muscles and tendons in my leg by polio and the surgeries I had while young simply complicate an already complicated situation. Dr. Syed and Vaiva don't give me timelines and predictions because they don't know. Learning to walk doesn't come with a manual or a service guide, and that's something else I am learning.

32

MY OLD COMPANION,
PAIN

I have a lifelong and deeply intimate relationship with pain. My account of my experiences at the Buddhist retreat is but a brief introduction to the pain I have experienced over the years and the ways I have reacted to it.

In our medicine cabinet is a bottle of PMS-Hydromorphone. According to one drug directory, "Hydromorphone belongs to the family of medications known as opioid analgesics (narcotic pain relievers). It is used to treat moderate to severe pain, including pain after surgery. High concentration injectable forms of this medication are only used to treat severe pain for people who need higher than usual doses of hydromorphone."

A doctor at Hillcrest Hospital gave me the bottle of PMS-Hydromorphone the day I was leaving to go home. I told her it was unlikely I'd use it; I had been weaning myself off the drug for the last week at the hospital and was relying more often on the extra-strength Tylenol that the nurses gave me in between doses of hydromorphone. The routine at the hospital was that you took painkillers before physiotherapy, late in the day and before going to bed. They also liked to give you sleeping pills before bed. I had stopped taking the sleeping pills in my first week, and in my last week I had tried to restrict my intake of hydromorphone to the moments after my physio when, and if, it appeared as if my leg would drive me to scream. The doctor at Hillcrest smiled and said, "Just take the pills home, they might come in handy. You need to be out of pain in order to concentrate on your healing and your physiotherapy." I think we each silently agreed to let the other live out their respective delusion: she didn't think there was any possibility I wasn't going to use the pills and I was convinced that in time the bottle would be thrown out without ever being opened.

During the first six months at home after surgery, I found a number of ways to cope with the pain created by the exercises and by the nerve repair process. For the exercise pain, heat and cold in appropriate measures and a personal massage wand for muscle tightness worked, as long as I didn't avoid meditation and sleep. For the nerve pains, I adopted a plan based on distraction. When the leg went crazy and the signals misfiring between the leg and the brain grew intense, I would lift weights. It was a fairly bizarre scene, Debi and I in the evening watching a bit of television and all of a sudden I would stand on one foot and do a series of arm lifts with a five-pound barbell. Then I would sit, watch a bit more TV and repeat. The weights had nothing to do with the leg, but a physician friend suggested it was all about releasing endorphins in the brain, a natural form of pain relief. Endorphins, distractions, a routine to concentrate upon are all useful in navigating one's way through a maze of pain. I had used variations of all three for decades.

What I didn't realize right away was that I was undergoing a significant change in my relationship with pain. It didn't really register for a few weeks. But one morning I woke up and realized as I lay there that I was suspiciously without pain. There's a body scan meditation that's an exercise in awareness, where you bring your focus of attention individually to the various parts of your body and check in, see how everything is going. You zero in on your foot, your ankle, your calf, your knee, etc., and you take the pulse, measure the mood and determine what if anything that part of you is signalling. As I started the body scan, I realized that what was truly different this morning was that I wasn't registering pain in any of my usual pain centres. I was simply lying in bed and enjoying the experience.

When I wake up in the morning now, I feel no pain. While falling asleep, I feel no pain. While driving in the car or sitting in a movie theatre or at a restaurant, I feel no pain. Pain has been my constant companion almost as long as I have been alive. Waking without pain, sleeping without pain, going about my day without pain are new experiences for me.

There had been clues before that early morning epiphany. For weeks after I had returned home from the operation and my stay in rehab, people had been telling me how relaxed and rested I looked. I just assumed it was because I was resting and sleeping more, and of course that was part of it. I realized, though, that the much bigger piece of this "Wow, you look great!" phenomenon was that my body was no longer dealing with or registering an almost all-encompassing and constant battle with intense pain.

The new normal is that, with the exception of some occasional pain in my hands from using the canes too much, and some temporary pain in the muscles of my left leg after working them too hard and making them do things they don't normally do, I am pretty much pain free. And thus, in my mind, pretty much normal.

"Pretty much normal" is exactly what I am trying to convey here. I am a sixty-year-old man with a sixty-year-old body that has definitely received more than its fair share of trauma. People my age feel aches, twinges, discomforts, dislocations and irritations. That comes with the territory. What I had been experiencing for almost my entire life was deeply gut-wrenching and often seriously distracting pain, which ranged far outside the territory.

Losing the pain has been liberating. I can concentrate more deeply, I sleep better, I have a sunnier disposition, I am more positive and patient and less anxious, and I have fewer lines on my face. Two years ago, intensifying pain was what had me most worried about my future. Even as I watched my body deteriorate, my walking grow even more problematic, it was the intensifying pain that worried me and had me perplexed as to how much more I could actually endure. All of that is gone.

There is no straightforward explanation for the pain vanishing. Dr. Syed, pleased by an unexpected outcome he would never have promised, observed that making a body even and straight has all kinds of unintended and unpredictable effects. My GP, when I discussed it with him, smiled and said, "Well then, whatever else happens, the surgery was worth it." That is true. I had expected that the insane pain that had been tearing me apart in the months before the surgery would be gone and that some of the other pain might be lessened, but the idea that my experience of pain would itself undergo such a revolution had never entered my mind. Ironically, this incredible reduction in the amount of pain I experience is the closest I have ever come to witnessing a miracle. I suspect it is not what my mother had in mind all those years she prayed to Saint Jude, but perhaps, as she believed, God does work in mysterious ways.

I am not an idiot when it comes to pain. I have learned a fair amount about it and have a good sense of what I can handle and where my limits are. I also know that there is a keen difference between chronic pain and the pain that comes from simply being alive and trying things. The chronic pain is the soul destroyer; the temporary pain in muscles and limbs that comes from relearning to walk is another, much more manageable story. The temporary pain is a marker that you are forcing the body, and within limits that's okay. At physiotherapy, after we have tried something truly different and perhaps very difficult, Vaiva always asks how the pain is and I always say, "It's okay, I can deal with it." It has become such a routine exchange that we both smile. It's only funny because it's true. A sore muscle from making the leg work is totally doable, easily endured.

In our medicine cabinet is a bottle of PMS-Hydromorphone. It has never been opened. God willing, it never will be.

33

MY NEW DAY JOB

You know the old joke when somebody shows you their writing or demonstrates their singing ability and they really aren't very good, and you respond, "Don't quit your day job"? In my case, quitting my day job in order to concentrate on what I wasn't very good at is just what I did.

Less than four months after my surgery, my health insurer wanted me to return to work. My surgeon thought it was a bad idea, Vaiva thought it was a crazy idea, but I figured I didn't have much choice. At this point I was still using crutches. Getting from point A to point B took time. Walks of any distance wore me out both physically and mentally.

I had worked at the CBC for a quarter of a century and loved my job for most of that time. Facing the tasks involved in getting my walking right for perhaps the first time in my life demanded of me a significant amount of physical and mental energy. While I still loved current affairs, was still an information sponge and was still enamoured of the stitching together of words and concepts, I knew that making sense of steps, understanding and altering my gait, exercising and utilizing long-dormant muscles, and just wrestling with the relatively mundane notions of where my foot was and what was my point of physical and mental exhaustion required making some tough decisions about priorities and necessities.

Physically accomplishing the return to work in January 2013 while still on crutches and still not competent at using the subway system meant Debi had to drive me, and that was not pleasant for either of us—not pleasant for me because I felt too much of a burden already, not pleasant for her because it meant navigating traffic both ways in the midst of morning and evening rush hours. Throw into the mix January weather, my need for physio twice a week, and just the sheer drag and anxiety wrapped up in the mundane but necessary chores of life, and the result is unhappiness.

Once at the office, life didn't get much simpler. The distance from the sidewalk outside the building to my office was for your average able-bodied guy a breeze; for a guy on crutches, less so. Crutches also meant no free hands, so everything I needed to bring to work or take to meetings required wearing a backpack, which is not an onerous task for most people, but for the guy on crutches it is just one more thing intruding on his consciousness when he's trying to walk. All the normal personal stuff that you take for granted in a working life—going for coffee, using the men's room, standing by a colleague's desk and chatting, or even preparing for a fire drill—become significantly more laden with decisions and difficulties when you are using crutches.

On top of all of this, there were the sheer mental demands of my work. I have always taken pride in my work, which was of a deeply cerebral nature. Lots of thinking, speculating, reading and talking with potential guests or experts for background information and analysis was the stuff of my every day. Coming up with story ideas and treatments as well as developing innovative approaches to both the serious and frivolous aspects of life constituted the expectation and norm of what I did for twenty-plus years.

The great British writer, journalist and aphorist Samuel Johnson once observed that "the prospect of being hanged focuses the mind wonderfully," and while I have never been in danger of having to undergo capital punishment, I do have a lived sense of what he was getting at. Concentrating on learning something as fundamental and foundational as walking gave me a real grasp of priorities. In the late fall of 2012, in the winter of 2013 and even today, getting walking right has taken up much of my time, attention and sense of perspective. What I have left of those attributes and skills I need to use wisely and on apt, right and worthy activities. As Johnson suggested, it wasn't so much that my other activities had lost their importance; they just weren't my priority any longer. Learning to walk yet again was making significant demands on my body, my mind and my will, and the reaction to these demands had to be proportionate. Something had to give.

In my years at the CBC I had acquired the right to a decent pension, Debi and I had some savings, and I had developed skills that were marketable in other fields. I realized that the time was right to make some real adjustments. Financially I was going to be okay, and professional work when needed would be possible, but at this moment change was in order. I was going to shift the focus of my energies from work to learning to walk, and with the time left over from that I would attend to family, and then, if and where possible, to work. I have long believed that the rightness of an idea or decision can be measured in the way it feels when finalized. The decision to leave the CBC felt right, timely and important.

Telling my colleagues was difficult. We had worked together for years and liked and trusted each other a great deal. For the most part the reaction was disbelief, a suggestion that my deciding to leave the CBC was something they had never expected.

That night, after Debi picked me up at work and we talked about my day and how the telling had gone, she and I went out for Vietnamese food in a small mall in our neighbourhood next door to a Shoppers Drug Mart where in the past few months I had bought a walker, some canes and a few other "mobility aid appliances." Over some sticky rice and fresh rolls, we marked a significant passage in my life. Knowing that I would be concentrating my energies and attention on my walking, imagining what that would mean for us in the months and years to come, helped re-create some of the true joy we had experienced in Vietnam the previous February. We weren't there yet by any means, but we could imagine it.

34

THE KINDNESS
OF OTHERS

I sometimes wake in the night, a much less frequent occurrence than it used to be. In addition to the normal nighttime reflections and regrets that preoccupy us all when alone in the dark, I often wrestle with the notion of being a burden. When Debi and Jane read this line, they will object and insist that it isn't the case, and I will believe them to be sincere, if perhaps overly polite. I don't wrestle with this concern out of some form of self-pity or in an attempt to make everything "all about me," but rather because the idea of being a burden influences everything we know and believe about health, wellness, individuality and humanity. If I have struggled with learning to walk correctly for decades, at the same time I have struggled with the idea, consequences and toll of being a burden.

One particular constant in this lifelong encounter with walking is my need for the help of others. Of course, that was obvious in my early years and even as a teen. I would not have survived, coped or thrived if it hadn't been for my parents and the numerous doctors, nurses, therapists and technicians whose offices, labs, operating theatres and gymnasiums I have availed myself of over the years. During my twenties and thirties, the assistance was subtler and was often about tolerance—friends, neighbours, co-workers and family who would come to my assistance, accept my moods, forgive my pain-related rudeness and simply and willingly, though occasionally resentfully, make accommodations as required by my handicap and hindrances. On the one hand, it is the normal give-and-take of life. On the other, when the person needing and receiving the assistance has a chronic condition, the demands and needs can far too often seem one-way and endless, with no possibility of reciprocation.

In the traditional wedding vows, reference is made to "in sickness and in health, in good times and in bad, and in joy as well as in sorrow," all of which is code for the deceptively simple and deeply demanding notion of "come what may." I witnessed the true complexion of "come what may" in my parents' relationship, and I realize just how demanding the burden can be for both parties. And I fear that I will be the burdensome one.

I have written that my mother is known in my extended family as a saint. While it is true that I had my difficulties with my father, it is possible that he hasn't received the credit, from any of his children, he deserved for the care he gave to my mother during the two decades over which she grew progressively more infirm. Ironically, given my own frequent impatience with my mother, I would often get angry with him for his lack of patience with her stiffness, her relative immobility, her pain and the ways in which her condition was somewhat responsible for the fact that their lives weren't what they had imagined they might be. Chronic conditions make everyone touched by the illness feel as if life to some degree isn't what it could have been.

When I was recovering from hip surgery, my initial "relative helplessness" and the demands it imposed landed primarily on Debi but also frequently on Jane. My recovery hasn't been speedy, but in some ways it has been marked by the milestones of reclaiming tasks and thus incrementally relieving Debi. At one of my regular meetings with Dr. Syed, I said I was doing pretty well in that the previous week I had been able to cook a meal and was now regularly emptying the dishwasher. Both Syed and the resident with him looked at me quizzically, as if to say, "That's your measure?" Accomplishing more and more of those daily chores remains my measure today.

35

ME AND MY GAIT

I don't clearly remember when I first heard the song "Me and My Shadow," the 1927 hit performed by Al Jolson and by numerous other performers over the years, but the central idea in the song—that a person and his shadow are inseparable and that where you find one, you find the other—has always struck a deep chord. In my case, it has never been so much about my shadow as my walk, and for years I have thought that if I were to rewrite the song I'd call it "Me and My Gait."

In the early 1980s, while I was studying law at Dalhousie University in Halifax, I took a part-time job at the Sir Frederick Fraser School for the Blind. On my first day of work, one of the staff took me to the children. It was seven in the evening, about an hour from bedtime. I was told the children were watching TV. I was taken aback for a moment and asked if that was really the case. I was assured that the kids liked TV, several were keen fans of *Hockey Night in Canada*, but almost all of them loved *The Dukes of Hazzard*. The staff person explained that hockey was one steady stream of play-by-play, so a blind child could follow along easily, while *The Dukes of Hazzard* was a show filled with explosions, noise, numerous mood-setting snippets of music, but most importantly a narrator who set up the premise of the episode at the beginning, and did a recap after every commercial and a wrap-up at the end. In other words, a perfect way to do television for the visually impaired and a precursor of today's described video.

When we arrived at the TV room, I was introduced to the children. I recall one very tiny girl, about seven, who, after being introduced to me, said with certainty that I "walked like a limp!" It took me a second to realize that audio cues were key to these kids and that when they heard someone walking the corridors, they used the speed, intensity, sureness and weight of the steps to make educated guesses about who belonged to what walking pattern. For all the time I worked at the school, the children referred to me as "Peter, who walks like a limp." It is a designation and descriptor that I have never forgotten and have been frequently reminded of over the past decade as I've started to read more and more articles about gaits and what a gait may or may not indicate. What those blind kids in the 1980s intuitively understood, doctors, profilers and all manner of professional and amateur psychologists are just now fully coming to grips with.

For the last half-dozen years, scientists and intelligence agencies in North America, Europe and the Middle East have been experimenting with recording technologies, surveillance cameras, satellite images and variations on facial recognition software to determine if it is possible to either track known terrorists or identify hitherto unknown terrorists simply by the way they walk. In the case of known bad guys, the theory is that one could build a bank of gait impressions, similar to fingerprints, and use the same to pick culprits out of a crowd. In the case of unknown bad guys, are there cues and suggestions in the way a person walks that might indicate states of mind, degrees of emotional turmoil or simply an unusual weight distribution that comes from wearing explosives, and which might give security officials a heads-up?

Canadian Security Intelligence Service (CSIS) agents trying to stop terrorists aren't the only people obsessed with developments in the field of gait analysis. Doctors are using gait assessments and especially gait deterioration as indicators of possible mental deterioration. Psychiatrists and psychologists assess gait as a possible indicator of depression, sadness or other debilitating emotional or mental states. At the BC Children's Hospital, in the Shriners Gait Lab, gait analysis is being used on young children to determine the nature of walking disorders and the type of intervention needed, everything from new braces to surgery. Gait analysis is also used as an analytical tool in cerebral palsy, muscular dystrophy and diabetes, and to distinguish between "elderly fallers and non-fallers."

Controversially, and from my perspective disturbingly, gait analysis is increasingly being used as a tool in employee hiring. All the folks who teach about body language and creating the best first impressions are now intent on using a gait analysis framework to give courses on how to impress potential employers. Walking fast might indicate you are a go-getter, walking at a steady pace might announce you are reliable and dependable, while walking erratically might suggest you are easily distracted.

Gait analysis is the new big thing in sports medicine and athletic training too, which stands to reason. For years, coaches have shot video of star performances and used it as a form of instructional manual for athletes intent on learning from the best. Coaches and athletes use whatever tools are available to enhance performance. Today we see labs and sports equipment companies offering gait analysis as a tool for selecting the perfect training technique and the ideal footwear. Heck, there are even gait analysis services for sporting dogs offered by the leading cutting-edge veterinarians.

It makes sense that gait analysis is all the rage. There is a belief, as that little girl at the Sir Frederick Fraser School for the Blind expressed thirty years ago, that if we can capture the essence of a person's gait, it will speak volumes about who they are, about their past, present and future. Aristotle, Leonardo da Vinci and even the French novelist Honoré de Balzac were keen students of the connection between gait and human personality. The study of gait worked its way into Balzac's novels and even a scientific paper, "Theory of Walking," which was both a description of and a prescription for "the correct way of walking." Balzac scholar Susana Collado-Vázquez argues that Balzac's understanding of the phases of gait is medically and scientifically accurate, as is his analysis of the factors that go into determining gait: "personality, mood, weight, profession and social class." Collado-Vázquez has written that the nineteenth-century writer came to his conclusions through observation and, as such, "in our technology-dominated times . . . serves as a reminder of the importance of observation."

I know that since the surgery my gait has changed and is changing. Debi, who has more opportunity to notice this than anyone else, frequently comments on how much different my walking is now than it was two years ago, a year after the surgery, before the surgery, and so on. My physiotherapist and her colleagues frequently comment on the significant differences they see in the way I walk from month to month. When I walk now, I stand tall instead of listing to one side. My stride is more confident and has less of a hitch. The weight distribution as I move is more even and my body in movement is slowly becoming more balanced.

In the literature about gait analysis, much is made of the possibility of changing one's gait through conscious effort. What's not clear is whether or not changing one's gait changes one's personality. I can attest to the fact that changing one's gait is possible if not easy, and my personality does seem to be changing. I am calmer, have a greater sense of equanimity, even increased patience. Are the changes I am noticing a result of no longer experiencing intense chronic pain, which is partly a consequence of having a body that is now relatively symmetrical? It is a chicken-or-egg dilemma that causes me to drift off into reflection.

In 2013, while in Rome with Debi, I spent some time at the Clinical Movement Analysis and Research lab of the Santa Lucia Foundation. One of the very bright minds who met with me was Yuri Ivanenko, who studies gait, gait development and gait pathology. Dr. Ivanenko is soft-spoken and displays a true scientist's reluctance to be 100 percent certain about matters still being researched. He has been studying gait for more than two decades and believes that what he has discovered is that there are always more questions and, perhaps more importantly and more surprisingly, that much of what we think we know about gait and how gait develops is speculative and uncertain.

At one point, while gesturing with his hands and enumerating how stance, hip movement, muscle arrangement, stride, posture, even the way one's hands move or don't move are all issues in gait description and development, he paused, shrugged, grinned slightly and suggested that maybe all we could do was approximate what gait was, how it develops and how it deteriorates. Before I could respond, he went on to say that he envied me because I had an insider's take on gait that he would never possess.

Since my surgery, I have spent more hours than I ever imagined observing my gait and other people's gait. It used to be that I abhorred plate glass windows and the evidence they gave me about my walk, but no longer. I seek out glass and mirrors as vehicles to judge how I am doing today. While it is not clear what my gait will ultimately be, I do know that, however I might describe it, I am now no longer "Peter who walks like a limp."

In February 2013, seven months after my surgery, Debi and I went to Palm Springs as part of our plan to escape the winter and enjoy the heat of the deserts of the southwestern United States. The idea was that I would get more used to walking in natural settings than was possible at physio sessions or inside shopping malls, museums and stores. From the moment we landed at LAX, we knew we had made the right decision. Being able to go outside without fear of snow or ice made it simpler for me to just walk. I found it easier psychologically as well, because Palm Springs is a community that has its fair share of folks using canes and walkers.

On our first full day in Palm Springs, we drove to a huge outlet shopping mall. For almost two decades, whenever I needed shoes, I went to one particular store and ordered one particular type of shoe and had it altered with a built-up heel. The range of shoes that can accommodate built-up heels is narrow. When I needed a built-up brace and shoes, I didn't so much shop for shoes as order my regular. The last time I had really shopped for shoes was before I broke my foot that last time, in the nineties. That was a time when going into a store and getting running shoes, desert boots or whatever caught my eye was as normal as going to a bookstore and choosing the book I wanted at that moment.

That day in the Rockport outlet shoe store, I walked up and down the aisles, mesmerized by the variety of types and colours. There were no limits on me other than the limits everyone faces: how large are my feet, how wide a shoe do I need. I pointed at a shoe and the store had my size. I sat down, tried them on, stood and looked at my feet in the mirror. I decided to take them and another pair I had been eyeing. As I stood at the cash and waited for my receipt, I thought, *Well, this is different. I could get used to this.*

EPILOGUE

My dreams are frequently about walking. Nightmares about walking gone terribly wrong; anxiety dreams about difficult walking; dreams where my walking is so fluid that I realize in the middle of the dream that it is a dream simply because it's going so well; dreams where I accomplish a stage of walking that I am struggling with; and sometimes, though rarely, dreams of running. These walking dreams are not new, though their frequency has increased since my hip surgery. Prior to my operation in August 2012, when I dreamt of walking, it was almost invariably about losing the ability to walk.

My mood when waking from the dreams varies. The pre-surgery dreams almost always left me in a foul state and often cast a pall over my day. The post-surgery dreams often leave me slightly sad, disappointed and frustrated that I have not yet perfected my walking. I have never been a perfectionist, but I have always felt the need to be better than I am; that my performance in any activity was inadequate, below par. I have learned that this is not uncommon among people who had polio, especially as very young children.

I am haunted by polio. In the months after my surgery, I was obsessed with stories about the outbreak of new cases, largely in war zones or in countries where civil society is collapsing. I had believed the repeated promises made during the 1990s and 2000s about the possibility and nearness of the eradication of polio. For a decade and a half, researchers have believed that it is possible, but as *New York Times* reporter Donald G. McNeil Jr. put it in a succinct summary of the efforts as of 2011, "getting rid of the last 1 percent has been like trying to squeeze Jell-O to death. As the vaccination fist closes in one country, the virus bursts out in another." Oftentimes, the "virus bursting out" is the result of politics, religion or geopolitical strategy putting the lives and futures of children on the sidelines in order to accomplish some other goal. I would sit in my room, forbidden to put weight on my leg, and rage silently at how easily we can lose sight of the goal of eradication and what a world without polio might actually mean. It is a disease that at its most serious cripples parts of the body and often the mind; in my case, it crippled my leg and left psychic scars on my personality.

My dreams sometimes cascade into what-ifs. If I hadn't developed polio, would they have caught the hip dysplasia? Would a Peter who didn't limp have been a different boy, a different man? Would not spending a year in a body cast in a small room at the back of a small house mean that today I would have different skills, a different perspective, a different life altogether? I have always found that the real problem with what-ifs is that the answers are both obvious and a fantasy. Life is what it is, and my life is my life.

Polio left me needing to prove myself. I am a stubborn man and find it difficult to be told I cannot do something. My experiences learning to walk for the third time have taught me that there are some things I cannot do, that I will never do, and that's okay. I'll never run, my foot drop will always be there, I will never be completely free of my cane. But I can walk, I don't limp much anymore, and I get stronger every day, and all of that is more than okay.

An old proverb holds that in order to truly understand someone, you need to walk a mile in their shoes. After learning to walk many miles in my own shoes three times, I am now finally understanding who I am.

ACKNOWLEDGEMENTS

Were it not for a score of doctors, nurses, lab technicians and orderlies, and all the people who keep hospitals, clinics and the health care system functioning and effective, I would not be alive and healthy today. Dr. Felix Klajner, my GP, and Dr. Khalid Syed, the surgeon who made my legs as they should have been, are just the latest in a long, long list of people I want to thank.

Learning to walk three times over the past six decades would have been truly impossible without the technicians who made my braces, fixed my shoes, adjusted my canes and explained to me so patiently and repeatedly just what I had to do in order to make my body move. And Vaiva Underys is a genius of a physiotherapist who deserves more credit than I can give for the way I walk today.

My family deserves true thanks for putting up with me when I was ill, dealing with the demands, both conscious and unconscious, that I made of the lot of them. My parents did not live to see me stand straight but I know it would have made them smile. My siblings have taken so much of my pain and difficulty in stride over our lives that I only hope they take some of the joy I feel today as their due.

The Random House of Canada family has been truly supportive and exhibited extreme patience with a writer who is not always keen on telling his own personal story. Anne Collins and Amanda Lewis prodded and poked me, stirred and encouraged me to open up fully on a journey that has been marked with sadness and joy, disappointment and real surprise. Scott Sellers, the publicity/communications wunderkind, has been very encouraging of the project since he first encountered me musing about my experiences. Random House of Canada is a joy to work with.

Two people have been such integral witnesses and provided vital aid and comfort during both my physical decline and my resurgence that even thinking about acknowledging them feels like thanking the air. My daughter, Jane, a wizard at words, has added so much joy and meaning to my being that I glow just thinking of the years we have known each other and smile in anticipation at the years to come. Debi, who taught me that I could be loved, makes me laugh, makes me think, and most importantly makes me the best person I can be.

As critical as all of these people have been in shaping who I am today, none of them is responsible for any of the things I have gotten wrong or misunderstood in the telling of this story. My mistakes, like my stumbles while walking, are all mine.

BIBLIOGRAPHICAL NOTE

Much of this memoir is based on memories, my own and others'. In order to make sense of my own experiences and the times I lived through, I read widely and generally about Deep River, polio and the history of orthopaedics, diagnostic medicine, surgical techniques, walking, muscle development, the functions of nerves and the construction of braces. Over the years I have read extensively in the areas of religion, pain and pain management, Buddhism, the psychology of self and the lasting effect of injury and insult on the human psyche. As with most of us, the combination of what I have lived and what I have learned has helped shape my world view, fashioning my sense of who I am and how I have navigated my life so far.

For details about polio and polio epidemics, I consulted materials from the Ontario Archives, the Hospital Library and Archives at the Hospital for Sick Children in Toronto, and the archives of the *Globe and Mail*, the *Toronto Star* and the *Toronto Telegram*.

I also consulted the medical website of the Smithsonian's National Museum of American History, and the websites of the Centers for Disease Control and Prevention, the Mayo Clinic, the Health Heritage Research Services and the World Health Organization.

The following books, articles and websites were of use in understanding the history of surgical techniques, gait, and how walking works and develops.

Collado-Vázquez, Susana (translated by J.M. Carrillo). "Balzac and human gait analysis." *Neurologia* (May 31, 2012).
Edwards, Glen E. and Douglas B. Harkness. *Life Near the Bone: A History of Orthopaedic Surgery in Alberta*. Our Roots: Canadian Local Histories Online, 1991.
Rose, Jessica and James G. Gamble. *Human Walking* (3rd ed.). Baltimore, MD: Lippincott Williams & Wilkins, 2009.

Among the sources for my reflections on Catholicism and Buddhism were the websites operated by St. Joseph's Oratory and the National Shrine of St. Jude, *Radical Acceptance* by Tara Brach (New York: Bantam, 2003), *Going to Pieces Without Falling Apart: A Buddhist Perspective on Wholeness* by Mark Epstein, M.D. (New York: Crown, 1999) and *Mindfulness Meditation for Pain Relief: Guided Practices for Reclaiming Your Body and Your Life* by Jon Kabat-Zinn (Louisville, CO: Sounds True, Inc., 2009),

NOTES

Specific quotations are as follows:

p. 18 "Give oxygen through the lower . . ." from Tony Gould, *A Summer Plague: Polio and Its Survivors* (New Haven: Yale University Press, 1997).

p. 28 "6 weeks: sits . . ." from Lawrence Miall, Mary Rudolf, Malcolm Levene, *Pediatrics at a Glance* (Malden, MA: Blackwell Science, 2003).

p. 39 "Jesus stepped into a boat . . ." Matthew 9:5, *New American Bible* (Rev. Ed.) (New York: Catholic World Press, 2011).

p. 40 "Brother André . . ." prayer to Saint Brother André, www.catholicdoors.com. Accessed November 10, 2014.

p. 46 "For physicians who were . . ." from Edwards and Harkness, *Life Near the Bone: A History of Orthopaedic Surgery in Alberta*.

p. 85 "Look at the patient . . ." by Dr. Richard Asher, quoted in Colleen S. Campbell, "Deconditioning: The Consequences of Bed Rest" (Institute on Aging, Department of Aging and Geriatric Research, University of Florida, 2011).

p. 94 "O glorious apostle . . ." Prayer to Saint Jude, http://www.ecatholic2000.com/cts/untitled-405.shtml.

p. 95 "O Holy Saint Jude!" Prayer to Saint Jude, http://www.ourcatholicprayers.com/prayer-to-st-jude.html.

p. 112 "I recall a patient of mine . . ." from "How do I use a cane?" Ask Doctor K, February 28, 2012, http://www.askdoctork.com/how-do-i-use-a-cane-201202281320.

p. 115 "Scarification (intentionally scarring a person's body) . . ." from "Scar Fashion," *Bizarre Magazine*, http://www.bizarremag.com/tattoos-and-bodyart/body-mods/5686/scar_fashion.html.

p. 115 "discovered a possible treatment . . ." from Miguel Perez-Aso, Luis Chiriboga and Bruce N. Cronstein, "Pharmacological blockade of adenosine A2A receptors diminishes scarring," *The FASEB Journal*, June 5, 2012, http://www.fasebj.org/content/early/2012/07/05/fj.12-209627.abstract.

p. 116 "at any age, bullying . . ." from Marie Ellis, "Bullying affects children's long-term health, study shows" *Medical News Today*, February 17, 2014.

p. 119 "Pain is not a punishment, pleasure is not a reward" from Pema Chödrön , *Comfortable With Uncertainty: 108 Teachings on Cultivating Fearlessness and Compassion* (Boston, MA: Shambhala, 2004).

p. 121 "When touched with a feeling of pain . . ." from "Sallatha Sutta: The Arrow," translated from the Pali by Thanissaro Bhikkhu, http://www.accesstoinsight.org/tipitaka/sn/sn36/sn36.006.than.html.

p. 122 "Physical pain is the response of the body . . ." from an interview between Joan Duncan Oliver and Jon Kabat-Zinn, "Pain Without Suffering," *Tricycle Magazine* (Winter 2002).

p. 123 "There is grace in suffering . . ." from Andréa R. Vaucher, "America's Guru," *Tricycle Magazine* (Winter 2013).

p. 129 "As the Buddhist view has consistently demonstrated . . ." from Mark Epstein, "Shattering the Ridgepole," *Tricycle Magazine* (Spring 1995).

pp. 143–44 "You gradually stretch out . . ." from Mollie Bloudoff-Indelicato, "New Limb-Lengthening Tech May Reduce Complications for Sufferers of Crippling Deformities," *Scientific American* (December 27, 2012).

p.183 "Hydromorphone belongs to the family of medications . . ." from C-Health Medi-Resource, Canoe.ca. http://chealth.canoe.ca/drug_info_details.asp?brand_name_id=1945

p.197 "personality, mood, weight . . ." from S. Collado-Vázquez, "Balzac and Human Gait Analysis".

PETER KAVANAGH is a veteran of Canadian media, having worked for twenty-five years at the CBC in television and radio with programs such as *The Journal*, *Morningside*, *The Sunday Edition* and *Ideas*, as well as publishing in the *Globe and Mail*, *Toronto Star*, *National Post* and numerous publications in the United States and Europe. He lives with his wife, Debi Goodwin, in Ontario.